The 28-Day Immunity Plan

The 28-Day
Immunity Plan

*A Vital Diet and Fitness Plan to Boost
Resilience and Protect Your Health*

ROSEMARY CONLEY CBE
WITH MARY MORRIS MSC

PENGUIN BOOKS

PENGUIN BOOKS

UK | USA | Canada | Ireland | Australia
India | New Zealand | South Africa

Penguin Books is part of the Penguin Random House group of companies
whose addresses can be found at global.penguinrandomhouse.com.

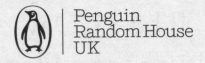

First published 2021
002

Text copyright © Rosemary Conley, 2021
Cover and exercise photography © Allan Olley, 2021

Food photography by Clare Winfield

The moral right of the author has been asserted

Set in 12.5/14.75 pt Garamond MT Std
Typeset by Jouve (UK), Milton Keynes
Printed and bound in Great Britain by Clays Ltd, Elcograf S.p.A.

The authorized representative in the EEA is Penguin Random House Ireland,
Morrison Chambers, 32 Nassau Street, Dublin D02 YH68

A CIP catalogue record for this book is available from the British Library

ISBN: 978–1–405–94912–5

www.greenpenguin.co.uk

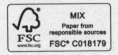

Penguin Random House is committed to a
sustainable future for our business, our readers
and our planet. This book is made from Forest
Stewardship Council® certified paper.

The information in this book is intended for general guidance only. While every effort has been made to ensure accuracy, it is not a substitute for and should not be relied upon as medical advice. Please consult with your GP or a qualified health professional to discuss possible modification of this programme to suit your specific health needs, and do not change, stop or start any treatment or medication without obtaining their advice. The author and publishers disclaim, as far as the law allows, any liability arising directly or indirectly from the use, or misuse, of the information in this book, or from any specific health needs that require medical supervision.

Contents

About the Authors

Rosemary Conley CBE is one of the UK's most successful diet and fitness experts with 50 years' experience helping people lose weight and get fitter. It all began with six of her neighbours meeting in her kitchen in 1971 learning how to slim down and make the most of themselves, and Rosemary has continued to take weekly classes ever since. But it was in 1988 that she shot to fame with her international best seller, *Hip and Thigh Diet*, which she wrote having lost weight on her hips and thighs after being recommended to follow a low-fat diet for medical reasons.

From 1993–2000 Rosemary appeared regularly on ITV's *This Morning*. From 1993–2014 Rosemary Conley Diet & Fitness Clubs operated throughout the UK. From 2014–2019 Rosemary was part of the team that ran Rosemary Conley Online. From 1996–2000 Rosemary was a Consultant to Marks & Spencer, advising them on their healthy food range.

Over the years Rosemary has captured the attention of the nation with her simple and effective diet and exercise plans. Her 36 books and 30 fitness DVDs have sold over nine million copies worldwide.

In 2004, Rosemary was awarded a CBE in the Queen's New Year Honours 'for services to the fitness and diet industries'. She appeared on BBC's *This is Your Life!* in 2002 and on ITV's *Dancing on Ice* in 2012. Rosemary was the first woman ever to be made an Honorary Freeman of the City of Leicester, and she is a Deputy Lieutenant of Leicestershire. Rosemary continues to have a high media profile with many regular appearances on national radio and television.

Mary Morris MSc originally trained as a PE teacher at IM Marsh College of PE in Liverpool and then taught in secondary schools for six years before starting a family. She never returned to the school playing fields however and instead developed her career into adult fitness, establishing Community Exercise classes in her local area.

It was in 1982 that she opened her own Health Club in Lichfield, which she ran for over 30 years in partnership with her husband.

In 1986 she was one of the founders of the RSA Exercise to Music qualification and became a Course Director for the Midlands, running training courses for the YMCA. She became Chief Verifier for the RSA Examinations Board in 1989.

Since 1994 Mary has worked with Rosemary Conley as a Teacher Trainer, Fitness Consultant and Choreographer of most of her fitness videos/DVDs, forming a successful working relationship that exists to this day.

In 2004 Mary gained her MSc Degree in Exercise and Nutrition Science at University College Chester and then went on to train as a fully qualified Pilates instructor. Mary has been teaching exercise for almost half a century and still runs community classes teaching Pilates, Strength Training and Aerobic sessions for older adults in her community.

Confronting Coronavirus

This is a simple 28-day plan to help boost your immune system no matter what your age, which also includes a workout that is specifically designed for the older generation. We will help you transform your fitness in a way you never thought possible and assist you in shedding unwanted weight fast! All in the comfort of your own home and without pain!

We all want to stay safe in these challenging times and it's not too late to make a real difference to our immune system and increase our chances of surviving the potentially fatal COVID-19 pandemic – or other infections or viruses. And it's easier than you think.

Whilst we are only too aware that the terrible coronavirus can hit anyone at any age, we are continually reminded that those most at risk from coronavirus are people who are overweight or obese (at the peak of the pandemic, 73 per cent of people admitted to ICU were overweight or obese and 80 per cent of deaths were people over 70). Others at higher risk are those suffering from asthma, heart disease and diabetes or who have compromised immune systems. Alarming statistics emerging indicate that patients who were overweight or obese were twice as likely to lose their battle with COVID-19, so it is really important that we learn from this.

But there is hope and that's what this book is all about.

No matter what our age, by taking some simple steps to change our everyday lifestyle – the way we eat, drink and exercise – we can dramatically improve our immune system, lose a few pounds and increase our fitness as well as our chances of living a longer, fitter and healthier life.

With a simple but highly effective healthy eating plan, which includes foods that specifically boost your body's natural defence system, we can also help you shift those unwanted pounds – particularly those you might have gained during the many lockdown months. And the progressive 28-day immunity-boosting workout will leave you astonished at how fast you can progress your fitness to become fighting fit!

All we ask is that you give us 28 days to help change your life for the better. We hope that the experiences of our trialists will inspire you into action. They transformed their lives by following the programme and have chosen to continue beyond those initial four weeks because of the enormous benefits they have personally experienced. We have loved reading their heartwarming comments and hearing how they have naturally adapted their lifestyle to what is now their 'new normal'.

If you follow the guidelines in this plan, you can not only improve your fighting power against COVID-19 and other viruses, but you will also feel so much better, both physically and mentally, and hopefully create some great new lifestyle habits for yourself and your loved ones for the future.

1. Tried and Tested

Over the decades of my writing many different diets I have always found it helpful – to me and to the reader – if my eating plans were put to the test with real-life trialists. Learning from the personal experiences of volunteers who have followed the programme always helps me to add, tweak or change any elements that can be improved, so that by the time the book is published, I feel completely confident in its effectiveness.

This book presented me with a wonderfully different opportunity to not only design an eating plan that would help followers lose a few pounds if they needed to, but, most importantly, that they would be able to *feel* a difference to their general health and well-being after following it for just 28 days. Rather than a 'diet' plan it is a 'health' plan. In this chapter, my trialists explain their experiences.

This book was originally written as an eBook, which was published by Penguin in August 2020. I wrote it when we went into lockdown at the end of March and I needed to turn it around quickly to ensure that it was published as soon as possible while the COVID-19 pandemic was still current. Little did we know then that the threat of this deadly virus would be around for so long, added to which we are consistently reminded by scientists that even if a vaccine for the coronavirus can be found, there will be other viruses around the corner. This whole experience has certainly given the world a new perspective on life. Never before, certainly in my lifetime, has there been such a desire to make lifestyle changes to help us live longer and healthier lives. This has to be good news because it motivates us to take positive action like never before and the rewards for so doing are, quite simply, tremendous.

When I started writing the eBook, I worked on the eating plan, recipes and the concept of what we needed to do to boost our immunity. I asked my co-author, Mary Morris, to design the section on fitness and an exercise plan that would work alongside it. Both Mary and I really hoped that the eBook would be sufficiently successful for the publishers to invest in taking the book into a paperback version. Whereas my trialists were a variety of ages from 32–74 years, Mary thought it would be a great idea to run a trial too, but this one would focus particularly on older and previously inactive participants taking up exercise for the first time for a good while. Because of the health risk to this age group from COVID-19, Mary wanted to see what difference could be achieved in 28 days to those who previously had lived a fairly sedentary lifestyle. The results proved fascinating and inspirational. You can read more on Mary's Trial in Chapter Seven.

You can imagine Mary's and my delight when the news came that Penguin had decided to take our little eBook to be published as a paperback early in 2021. We immediately set about enhancing the original version and expanding it, otherwise this would have been a very slim book!

In this new and updated version, as well as lots more

information on nutrition I have included additional meal choices, plus some extra recipes, whilst Mary has added more exercises. In the original version the workout was designed specifically for the older generation but, despite that, my trialists really enjoyed it and found great benefit from adapting the exercises to their fitness ability. In this new version of the book, Mary has designed an additional workout that will be suitable for *all* ages.

In this chapter I would like to introduce you to my own Trial Team and to share with you their experiences of following the Plan.

First, I must introduce them. Since 1971 I have run slimming and exercise classes in Leicester and the only time, apart from holidays or for medical reasons, I have had a break from the classes was for six months when I was on *Dancing on Ice* in 2012. Taking my classes is an absolute joy and meeting with my group every week is a privilege and a pleasure and I consider them to be my friends. Many have been attending for over 30 years, and some for over 40, with a dozen of them now in their 70s and five in their 80s! Their ongoing fitness is due in no small part to their dedication in attending those weekly exercise sessions.

When we had to suspend the classes because of COVID, we formed a private WhatsApp group where my members were able to keep in touch and we could share our ups and downs of self-isolation, restricted movement and pictures of our gardens or the views from our regular walks. We have become an even closer friendship group as a result, which has been one of the bonuses of these strange times.

The day after I heard that Penguin was going to publish our eBook, in the hope that it would ultimately be published in paperback, I emailed my WhatsApp members explaining that I was looking for volunteers for a trial. Within a day, Brigitte, Helen, Dawn, Lesley, Jennie and her son Kevin, Mike and Michelle came forward. I set them up with the Plan from my raw manuscript and asked them to put The 28-Day Immunity Plan to the test.

It made me smile when I heard that when the email arrived in Brigitte's husband's inbox, Dave turned to her and said, 'You need to do this!' For Brigitte, like so many, the lockdown had meant there was a bit more snacking going on and waistlines were expanding.

It is important to understand that The 28-Day Immunity Plan is not a 'diet plan' but a 'health plan'. I asked the Trial Team to text me each week with their observations and weight losses if they had any, and I called them every Monday night to check how they were feeling. At the end of the 28 days I asked them to complete a questionnaire and this is what they said:

Weeks 1–4

Lesley (age 59)

'I am so pleased! I am sleeping better and don't feel so bloated or sluggish. I love the fact that I could eat as much salad and veg as I wanted. It was so simple to follow. I feel *better*, and more positive about my weight control. I have definitely found my "get up and go". I feel *cleaner* on the inside. I *want* to get on the scales instead of dreading them! I love the simplicity of the Plan. I don't have to count calories or weigh food – just use my common sense.

'I've lost 2 inches off my waist and an inch off my hips. I love the fact that the rules are very clear. I know what I can eat and what is off limits because it's unhealthy. That suits my personality and really helped me to stay focused. I have totally changed the way I think about food now because I feel so good in myself and I will continue eating this way going forward.' (*In the 28 days Lesley lost 8lbs*)

Helen (age 49)

'I was at such a "low" in lockdown and being on my own meant that I was feeling miserable and lonely. This Plan came along at exactly the right time. I never thought I would lose as much weight as I did and was pleasantly surprised by the increase in my energy levels and how much better I feel in myself overall, which in turn has made me a happier person.

'The greatest benefits to me were greatly improved sleep; eating three healthy meals a day at normal times, which I haven't done for a long time; my energy levels have increased greatly and I am waking up more alert and with a spring in my step! Also, I don't appear to have any stomach/bowel problems any more – *and* I've lost weight!

'I am pretty active anyway because of the horses, but I benefitted from the exercises in the Plan. It made me realise that my legs were not as strong as I thought they were and I like the fact that the exercises worked my entire body.

'For me, this was an "improved way of eating" rather than a diet. I love having more energy and the desire to do more and I have never slept so well for years! I will definitely continue to eat in this new way because I feel great!' *(Helen lost 11lbs)*

Dawn (age 56)

'I joined the Trial as I wanted to lose some weight and become fitter. At the end of the four weeks I felt "better" and "healthier" in myself and my skin was clearer too and I slept *so* much better! I found the portion sizes were enough for me and I bulked out with salad and vegetables when I needed to.

'Because of recent foot surgery, I cycled rather than walked every day at the beginning but lapsed a bit in Week 3 due to the weather. I was surprised at how strenuous the workout that's included in the Plan turned out to be, but I enjoyed seeing my progress in being able to increase my reps compared with when I started. I'm pleased with my progress.' *(Dawn lost 7.25lbs)*

Brigitte (age 62)

'When I started on the Trial I wanted to get myself back on track. I found coping with the coronavirus concerns that were going around caused my anxiety levels to be really challenging and I didn't want to feel sluggish any more. My snacking habits had taken over and my normal "routine" had disappeared. I just wanted to feel physically stronger and healthier.

'Biscuits have always been my downfall – in-between meals and snacking in the evening – but I HAVE COMPLETELY CUT THEM OUT! I cut down alcohol allowing myself just 1–2 small glasses of wine on a Friday and Saturday evening.

'After 28 days I feel proud to say that I am in a really good place. I am blown away with my weight loss – really amazed myself that I've done this just by sensible exercising and eating healthily. I feel good in my clothes, I feel happier, I feel much stronger, more energetic and I'm not feeling tired. I am totally confident that I will carry on with this new way of eating and activity going forward.

'The biggest change will be stopping eating in-between meals. I enjoyed the exercises and they really worked for me. I definitely feel stronger in my core, my legs and my posture and my energy levels are oh, so much better! I "want" to do things rather than thinking "I need to do . . ."

'I was surprised how easy I found it to follow the Plan and how quickly I loved getting into all the exercising routine and how good I was feeling. I was waking up feeling so refreshed from a good night's sleep. I don't feel tired, the bloated feeling has gone, I feel well and I don't feel sluggish any more – and I've lost 2 inches off my waist!

'This has been such a personal goal, not only for my personal self-esteem but I wanted to prove to myself that I could focus and achieve this goal for *me*. Now, I am really proud of myself and I feel oh so much better!' *(Brigitte lost 7lbs in the 28 days)*

Mike (age 32)

(Mike first joined my class with a school friend when they were both 14 years old. They lost weight and were such good movers in the exercise class that I selected them to appear in one of my fitness videos and, later, Mike was selected again to appear in one. I have seen him go through University, qualify as a graphic designer and even buy his own house. Except when he was at Uni, Mike has continued to attend my classes to help him stay on track.)

'I needed a kick up the bum to get my mind back into eating healthily and losing weight. Joining the Trial and following the Plan helped me focus on myself again and made me feel better – so much better – mentally and physically.

'I had got into the habit of nibbling a few treats in the evenings, which I've stopped, but if I really had a craving for something sweet, I would have a small portion of natural yoghurt and honey.

'I felt really positive about myself, which I hadn't felt for a while, which then made me feel I could come out the other side of the current COVID situation – losing weight and feeling good rather than putting weight on and feeling crap!

'I loved that the Eating Plan gave me the freedom to have unlimited salad as it made me feel like I'd eaten enough but I knew it was good for me and wouldn't impact on my losing weight.

'The greatest benefit was feeling better about myself and getting my head back on track so that I could continue to lose weight and eat healthily. I am now a stronger version of myself. I feel better mentally and physically, and generally more positive. It's given me the kick up the bum I desperately needed. It's reminded me to take care of myself and what I need to do in order to do that. I have realised that it is really important that we should all rethink what we put in our mouths so that we can stay healthy.' *(Mike lost 8.5lbs)*

Jennie (age 74)

(Jennie had already lost 5 stone at my classes and has suffered with severe back issues for many years, but she has found coming to the classes beneficial both physically and emotionally.)

'I adore lattes and normally have several every day, but since I started this Plan I have cut them out completely. I have enjoyed the walks and following the Eating Plan and eating so many different vegetables – and I am delighted with my weight loss. I knew I had gained weight over lockdown – a good 4lbs – and I needed to do something. I am very pleased with myself.

'One of the greatest benefits has been losing weight with my son, Kevin, who lives with me. We have enjoyed trying the different recipes in the Plan and we have been out walking together every day. I also did as many of the exercises as I could, bearing in mind my physical restrictions.

'I am amazed at how much weight I lost. In the first week I lost 7lbs, then 1lb, then another 2lbs and in Week 4, I lost 5lbs! I have more energy now and feel fitter, knowing what exercises I can do. I feel so much healthier and I am determined to keep eating well and to keep healthy.' *(Jennie lost 1 stone 1lb)*

Kevin (age 54 – Jennie's son)

'I decided to give it a go for two main reasons – firstly, because I had put on a little weight and wanted to get back down, and secondly, to support my mum. I enjoyed spending time and supporting her on the Trial and eating more healthily generally. I found the portions of the menus were generous and I intend to continue to experiment with various ways of cooking more new recipes. Whilst I have the occasional treat, I eat much more healthily now and certainly avoid some foods.

'I feel fitter and have greater endurance when I exercise, being able to keep going for longer and feeling less tired afterwards. I enjoyed going for a daily walk with Mum and I have lost 4 inches off my waist.' *(Kevin lost 1 stone)*

Michelle (age 55)

(Halfway through the Trial Michelle had to go into hospital for a small operation, which inevitably meant she was physically restricted for a while and unable to exercise. She recovered well and soon managed to get back on track.)

'My main reason to join the Trial was to lose weight and I liked the fact that I could eat unlimited salad and vegetables because I love those anyway.

'I felt this was a great Plan to give you a kickstart and get you back on track after all the anxiety caused by the coronavirus situation. I am delighted with my 2 inches lost from around my waist and interestingly, I feel lighter on my feet. I feel so much better in myself.' *(Michelle lost 10.5lbs on the 28-day Trial)*

At the end of the 28 days, my eight trialists had each lost an average of 10lbs and transformed the way they felt inside and out: their health, their energy levels, their sleep, their confidence – in fact, they had transformed their lives! I was so proud of them.

Weeks 5–12

Imagine my surprise when, at the end of the 28 days, every single one of my trialists asked if they could carry on. I was happy to continue keeping in touch and monitoring their progress, in fact, I welcomed the opportunity. COVID-19 was still very much present and I didn't want the anxieties and stresses of these challenging times to cause them to fall by the wayside. As so often happens after a trial, when the incentive and motivation of the Trial has past, it is so easy for old habits to creep in. My aim was to help them to achieve a 'healthy' BMI of less than 25.

Whilst I was delighted that they were determined to continue, I emphasised that I would be totally happy if they were able to just maintain the weight they had lost on the Trial. That in itself would be a great result. I also explained that if they were able to continue for two more weeks, their new eating and fitness regime would then become a lifestyle habit – their 'new normal' if you like – as six weeks of trying something new is recognised as the length of time needed to 'reprogramme' our brains and lifestyles into new habits.

As the weeks passed, the COVID restrictions started

lifting and life was beginning to return to something like normality in certain sectors, albeit with adaptations and changes to comply with social distancing measures and wearing masks. Some were returning to work, schools were reopening and restaurants and pubs were opening again. Four of my trialists work in the education system and life was getting busier. Despite this, they were determined to stay focused and to eat healthily and exercise as much as they could fit in.

My trialists reached the six weeks and just carried on! At the end of a further six weeks, now 12 weeks since they started the Trial, I asked everyone to complete another questionnaire. This is what they said:

Lesley

'I have loved it! It was so liberating for me not to have to worry about the portion size – if I was hungry, I added more vegetables. It suddenly dawned on me how much my energy levels had increased. A few days ago, I was even attempting to play football with my grandchildren! Before the Trial, I would have been on the sidelines watching them play and not even considering joining in!

'The other day I was sitting at my dressing table when I glanced down and thought, "My goodness! My thighs look thinner!" I hadn't really noticed until then. Then I tried on a dress that I hadn't worn for ages because it was too small and now it fits! I remember the first time I wore it was for my granddaughter's 7th birthday. She will be 12 next month! I feel I have "undone" five years of nibbling . . . yay!

'My bloated feeling has completely gone and I still feel

cleaner on the inside and my energy levels just keep increasing. I notice I am walking quicker without getting out of breath and when I walk uphill, I no longer have to stop to catch my breath. I am so proud of myself! I feel like a new "me". Then, to cap it all, the other day I saw a friend I hadn't seen for six months. Her opening words were, "You look fantastic! What have you done?" I am so happy to be where I am now.

'My advice to anyone thinking of following this Plan is to declare to your household that you want to do this for 28 days and you want and need their support. For those 28 days, make it your main focus as best you can and don't think beyond it. When you have got through it, you will want to keep going! It is the best thing I have done in years and it has changed my life!

'I realise that as a society we are going through a terrible time. I *used* this time to do something positive to improve *my* life as I approach my 60s, and with the sacrifices we are all making to keep each other safe, I feel this has been so worth it. People often lose weight when they have a medical scare, but COVID-19 has presented us with the best "medical motivation" we could have. Let's not waste it.' *(Lesley lost 1 stone 7lbs overall and now has a healthy BMI of 23.1)*

Helen

'Since the Trial, and the success I have seen in myself, I feel like I'm walking tall and starting to love myself and my body again. Since the start of the coronavirus pandemic I have worked from home and after a number of weeks this started to affect me mentally and physically. I was starting to withdraw into myself. Like many people, I felt lonely, isolated and unhappy.

'Having a healthy diet and exercise plan helped me to focus on looking after *me* and I was really surprised that a change in my diet would greatly improve my quality of sleep, mental health and general well-being, as well as give me so much more energy.

'Now I feel so much better in myself. It's sometimes easy to slip back into bad ways, but I find I *want* to eat healthily because I enjoy the food options on the Plan. In the middle of all this I had my 50th birthday and even though I gained a few pounds, I soon lost them again. I'm cooking a lot more with fresh ingredients instead of using convenience foods. I feel my entire body has been cleansed from the inside, which I'm sure is reflected on the outside. As someone who has suffered with stomach problems for years, I can honestly say this plan has helped far more than anything else I have tried.

'Never in my wildest dreams did I think that I would lose a stone, find new levels of energy, feel so much better in myself and maintain the motivation to continue. I am so glad that I volunteered and if people are serious about losing weight and feeling healthier inside and out, then I would 100 per cent recommend this Plan.

'Every part of me has benefitted. The best feeling is having more "get-up-and-go" in the mornings, enjoying better quality sleep and feeling healthier both on the inside and out. I have continued to work throughout the coronavirus lockdown but have still found time in the evenings and at weekends to clear out my house and create myself a little garden haven. This is something I haven't done for many years as I've always made excuses because I just didn't have the energy or motivation.

'Mentally I feel so much healthier, I am happier in myself and I know my confidence has increased. I now walk tall and stride out, with my head held high. I feel like a new me and I'm very proud of myself!' *(Helen lost a stone overall and now has a healthy BMI of 23)*

Dawn

'I felt much better in myself. I slept better and had more energy since following the Plan. I liked the fact that the menus were planned yet I could "pick 'n' mix" what I wanted – also the unlimited salad suited me.

'As the lockdown eased, eating out and BBQs have galloped back into my life – along with wine!

'I follow the Plan if we're not eating out during the week, but tend to fall off at the weekends now. When I was sticking to it, I felt *so* much better – I now need to organise my life more so that I can make time to plan and exercise. I followed the exercise plan initially, but my day job and my self-employed work have got in the way more recently.

'I'm not a morning person at all but when I was following the Plan it was definitely easier to get out of bed! Writing this, I've realised that I really do need to get back on it as I don't feel nearly as good now as I did after the initial 28-day Trial.' *(Dawn has lost 6.25lbs overall)*

Brigitte

'I feel really proud of myself. I'm glad I took the challenge of the Trial seriously and stuck to it and I have achieved very pleasing results. In Chapter One of the original eBook you said "You will be astonished at how fast you progress". Well, you do, and I proved that! I'm fitter, stronger, healthier and I sleep well! Because I have eaten so healthily and stuck to the rules of this Plan, I actually "feel" a big improvement to my immune system as well as my general well-being. I've made exercise fit in with me before work, which has become a normal routine for me now.

'I was a big biscuit eater and I missed them big time at the beginning but not any more. I completely cut them out in the 28-day Plan and even now, two more months later, I see them as a very occasional special treat and amazingly it doesn't bother me, plus I've stopped bingeing – thank goodness – and alcohol is now for weekends only and that's OK too.

'Having lost a stone and a good two inches off my waist, I feel so much better in myself and have so much more energy, plus I have received some lovely compliments on how I look. This Plan is now the new normal for me as I love the unlimited portions of vegetables and salad. They fill me up so that I really don't need "seconds" any more – which was another downfall of mine.

'I feel there have been so many benefits from doing this during lockdown. It's provided a great focus mentally, which has been helpful as we are all living life differently now. It has made me concentrate on my own health and fitness as I'm not getting any younger.

'I have really enjoyed the workout, which I have done from Day 1. What I loved was the gradual build-up to Week 4, which is what I follow now going forward. I have a set routine that has become a normal routine and I always do my 30-minute walk every day.

'It's great that any feeling of being bloated has gone and I don't feel sluggish any more. Yes, it's tough at the beginning as any new challenge is, but *do* challenge yourself and stick with it and do it for *you*, you will certainly enjoy and love the benefits.

'I will recommend this Plan to anyone to make them feel good about themselves again. The biggest thing personally is that I never came across any negatives. The whole experience has given me a real boost and a wake-up call! Thank you for getting me back into a really healthy lifestyle!' *(Brigitte now has a healthy BMI of 22.3)*

Mike

'As I'm sure many people did, during the first few weeks of lockdown I put on a bit of weight and was avoiding wearing my tighter-fitting clothes. Doing the Trial worked for me and I managed to drop the weight that I had initially put on plus more, so I was relieved when I felt it was safe to put on my "normal" clothes again and not feel like the buttons would ping off!

'I'm always beating myself up about my weight and I don't always feel good about myself but doing this Trial really helped me. Eating more healthily and committing myself to doing exercise, and being more active generally, definitely has made me feel better. It has improved my self-confidence and therefore makes me a whole lot happier and more positive.

'At the start of lockdown I was buying lots of treats and snack foods as I didn't know when I would be able to do the next food shop and I know I am prone to having cravings. The good news is that I don't tend to stock up on treats any more and if I do buy the odd "naughty", it's only a one-off and I definitely think twice before I stuff it in my face. I tend to ask myself: "Is this worth it? What good is this going to do for me and how nutritious is it?"

'I think I had got into the habit of eating the wrong things because of the new scary situation we were all in – not seeing friends and family and not being able to go out in public – so I felt like I didn't need to make much of an effort. My hair was growing out of control, so I didn't think it really mattered if my belly grew too! So, cutting back was hard to begin with but it also made me realise how much crap I was eating and that I really didn't need it.

'Eating more salad and veg as part of my meals is now the norm for me. I don't drink very often anyway, but I would say that questioning the things I put in my mouth is a big change for me as I would normally "eat now and regret it later"!

'Whilst I didn't follow the exercise plan, I did make myself do one of my fitness DVDs at least 2–3 times a week. I was also more active in general – instead of sitting on my backside watching Netflix! I walked much more and walked to the shops rather than drive. Somehow walking seemed to become more valuable during lockdown and I actually really enjoyed it.

'Following the Plan has made me aware of where I was

going wrong and how I could put it right. I realised that I needed to protect myself from the inside to help fight what was going on on the outside. The greatest benefit I have felt from doing the Trial is that I would say my mental attitude has changed for the better as I'm liking myself more. Having more self-confidence is a massive benefit.

'I'm really happy that I have lost even more weight than I lost during the 28-day Trial. I have now joined a gym for the first time in a few years, which I feel is a really positive result emerging from doing the Trial. I realise I need to push myself a bit further and pick up the slack, so joining the gym is a really important step for me and now I have the confidence to do it.' *(Mike lost 10lbs during the Trial)*

Jennie

(Please remember that Jennie had already lost 5 stone prior to the COVID lockdown.)

'The greatest benefit to me from this Plan was the fact that I am less bloated. I loved eating loads of vegetables and I felt there was plenty to eat, so I was never hungry and I feel very confident that I will carry on eating this way. I feel a lot healthier and much fitter.

'Prior to going on the Plan, I was addicted to lattes! During the 28-day Trial I cut them out completely but now I only have them as a very special treat!

'I've enjoyed my daily walks with my son Kevin, and we have enjoyed cooking the different recipes from the Plan together. It has been helpful doing the Trial together and we are really pleased with how we have each lost over a stone. I have much more energy and confidence, which is a real bonus. I'm sleeping better too.' *(Jennie lost 1 stone 4lbs on the Plan and now has a healthy BMI of 22.1)*

Kevin (Jennie's son)

'When I started on the Plan I weighed 16 stone 4lbs. Now, three months later, I weigh 14 stone 13lbs, which is not bad for my height of 6 feet 2 inches. My target was to get under 15 stone and I did it! I also lost 4 inches off my waist.

'The greatest benefits, as well as feeling better because of the weight loss, is I feel I am able to make better decisions about what and when I eat and I feel fitter and have much more stamina. I have enjoyed going for walks with Mum.

'If I feel hungry between meals, I now manage to hold out much more and I try really hard not to snack. If I feel I *have* to eat something, at least now it is something healthy. I have definitely cut my portion size down.

'I enjoy chocolate and used to eat it a lot more than I do now, eating some when I felt I needed a sugar boost, but now I find other alternatives instead. If we had a box of chocolates or chocolate biscuits in the house, it would have lasted a day or two once opened, but now it will last a week or two, or even longer.

'I very rarely drink, so I didn't miss alcohol. I love baking cakes but the last time I made one was for Mum's birthday last March!

'I have enjoyed looking at the recipes in the Plan and modifying them to our taste and we have explored different ways of cooking. We've tried new things too – like quinoa and sweet potato roasts. We've really enjoyed experimenting.

'Neither of us felt that we were following a "diet" but more a "guide to healthy eating". We both feel very confident that we will continue to eat this way going forward.

'Because of some stressful situations that I have had to deal with during lockdown, I feel that the fact that we have eaten healthily, and that I am so much fitter with more stamina, I have coped much better with stress during the difficult days.' *(Kevin lost 1 stone 4lbs and only needs to lose a little more to be able to fall into the 'healthy' BMI range)*

Michelle

'The other day I saw a reflection of myself in a shop window and it was much better! I used to be cross with myself when I saw my reflection, but not now – I like what I see! I've lost two inches off my waist and I feel lighter on my feet, I feel more energetic and not as fatigued as I was before the Plan. Even though I am a really light sleeper, I did sleep a bit better too.

'Alcohol wasn't a problem for me as I hardly ever drink, but I do miss having my normal desserts, but that's all. I feel better mentally as I feel more in control and I feel stronger in myself. I have had a couple of people ask if I've lost weight, which was great. Someone said my hair looked healthier too and I feel it's a bit thicker and in better condition.

'I enjoy doing my daily walks and some of the exercises

when I can, and I definitely feel healthier. I feel cleaner on the inside and more energetic generally.

'I'm really glad I did the Trial as it has meant that I am a stone lighter than at the beginning of the COVID crisis. I've lost 3 inches off my hips and I feel really well for it. I am really proud of myself.' *(Michelle now has a healthy BMI of 23.3)*

And finally . . .

Just as I was completing writing this book last September, on the day 'The Rule of 6' became law in England, I was chatting to my trialist Lesley just for a catch-up and she told me something that I would like you to hear. I asked her to write it down and here it is:

'We had gone to enjoy watching the football together but when we realised that this would be the last afternoon we could spend with all four grandchildren at the same time, Lauren [*Lesley's daughter*] suggested we stayed a little longer and she would do a little buffet.

'Normally, in this situation, I have a fight with that "little voice" in my head that tells me "start the diet again tomorrow", usually just the excuse I need to pile the buffet food high on my plate. That's OK if it's an isolated event but the problem is that when tomorrow comes, and I am faced with temptation again, it's easier to give in because I have already broken my resolve the day before anyway!

'But on Sunday, without thinking about it and for the first time *ever*, instead of saying "start again tomorrow", I kept saying, "*don't undo yesterday*". And I didn't! I had treats but I was realistic about what was sensible and I was never tempted to return for more. It's my new mantra – *Don't undo yesterday!*

As I am sure you can imagine, I am so proud of my Trial team and I hope their experiences will encourage you to give this Plan a go. As I have said earlier, try not to think of it as a 'diet and fitness plan', rather that it is a 'health' plan – a lifestyle-change programme that could save your life! And the bonus is that it will help you to live a longer, healthier and happier life. Surely that's worth working for, isn't it?

2. How to Boost Immunity in 28 Days

Eating healthily and keeping our weight under control is important at any age, but never more so than now. And if we are older, statistically we are at even greater risk of falling victim to coronavirus, so taking action now could be critical.

A good place to start is for us to look at ourselves in the mirror or get on the scales and face the facts.

Being overweight (that is having a BMI over 25), puts us at greater risk of heart disease, suffering a stroke, cancer, developing diabetes and now, much more. For those of us who are getting older, if we are overweight our joints begin to show the signs of wear and tear. In addition, our muscles are likely to become less strong because we are less active. Carrying around any 'excess baggage' can be both exhausting and depressing, as well as dangerous for our health – and if we store our fat around our middle (called visceral fat), this can put us at even greater risk.

Being overweight or obese is something that can be managed. Acknowledging that we *are* overweight is an important first step, but it is important that we don't use age as an excuse for carrying a few extra pounds. But there is great news! If we are able to transform our weight *and* activity levels, there is a significantly greater chance of our living a longer, fitter and healthier life.

Maximising the Results

The most effective and efficient way to boost our immunity is to eat foods that help to maximise the health of our white blood cells. These are the cells that fight infection and they are produced in our bone marrow.

The white-blood-cell-boosting foods include plenty of protein, some good-quality carbohydrate, a small amount of unsaturated fats and plenty of fruit and vegetables.

This immune-boosting weight-loss plan is full of these valuable nutrients. The menus created for each day will satisfy your appetite, and whilst you will also be cutting back on the calories, I don't think you will notice it. Whilst reducing calories is essential to create weight loss, it is also important for any diet to provide sufficient calories to meet our basic metabolic needs, and this eating plan does exactly that. If we put into our body 'immunity-boosting' fuel (food) and then raise our energy-spend by increasing our activity, we will maximise our ability to draw on our fat stores. Result? We lose weight and inches *and* boost our body's defence system. It can also help improve our mental health. It really is a win–win situation.

Our fat stores are like a 'savings account' of calories. Because we will be giving our body fewer calories than it burns in our everyday lives, the body *has* to find those extra calories from somewhere. When we exercise on top of that, we burn even more calories, so our body draws on our fat stores around our body to meet the shortfall. Not only do we lose weight and inches, we also reduce our fat stores, which is highly beneficial to our heart health and to our immune system. Exercising also boosts our immunity as it helps the lymphatic system to work more efficiently, which is key to the health of our infection-fighting white blood cells. You can read more about this in Chapter Six.

Foods to Boost Our Immune System

Protein

This is a vital component of white blood cells, so we need to eat a diet rich in meat, fish, eggs, cheese, yoghurt, milk and vegetables. If you follow a plant-based diet, ensure that you eat sufficient plant-based protein, such as quinoa, soy, beans, wholegrains and seeds. A vital mineral for our immune system is zinc, and this is found particularly in protein foods such as red meat, seafood, milk, beans, nuts, seeds, wholegrains, tofu and quinoa.

For our heart health particularly, aim to eat two portions a week of oily fish, such as salmon, mackerel, pilchards, sardines or herring.

Carbohydrate

This includes bread, cereals, pasta, rice and potatoes. Carbohydrate is needed for energy, so should be included – but in moderation – and it is important that we are selective in our choices. Try to eat wholegrain bread, high-fibre cereals, pasta, basmati rice and sweet potatoes, or new potatoes with skins, as these are more nutritious,

higher in fibre and are best for our all-important gut
health.

Unsaturated fats

These are found in a variety of oils, including olive, rapeseed, sunflower and safflower oil. They can help us absorb
fat-soluble vitamins such as vitamin D (which we get
from sunshine, and oily fish, such as mackerel, sardines,
salmon. In a plant-based diet, it can be found in fortified
oat, soy or almond milk) and vitamin A (which can be
found in fruit and vegetables and in plant-based foods).
Vitamin A is also an antioxidant that is important for our
health. We don't need a lot to make a valuable contribution to our immune system.

Vegan and vegetarian

With more and more people turning to eating a meat-free
or plant-based diet for humanitarian or environmental
reasons, the range of nutritious foods for this sector has
increased dramatically. There is significant evidence that
eating a plant-based diet is very good for our health as
these foods are more natural, but eating a plant-based diet
requires effort to ensure sufficient protein, vitamins and
minerals are consumed. Valuable plant-based protein
sources include lentils, chickpeas, almonds, quinoa, chia
seeds and hemp seeds. Beans and rice eaten on their own
are incomplete protein sources, but eaten together they
become a complete protein source.

Vitamins, Minerals and Supplements

We all need a variety of vitamins and minerals for our general health, but it is challenging to ensure that we have enough of everything we need to stay healthy and to fight infection. Supplements may have a role to play, but we have to be wary of false claims when it comes to products purporting to boost our immune system. Whilst the ideal is to absorb all of the nutrients we need naturally from the food we eat, that isn't always possible.

Vitamin C plays a particularly important role in fighting infection and we can enhance our immune system by eating fruit and vegetables every day. Lots of other micronutrients are also vital to our good health and if we are not always able to shop regularly, or we follow a restricted diet, sometimes we can become deficient in important vitamins and minerals and supplements can be helpful. When following any weight-reducing diet, even one as healthy as this one, it makes sense to protect ourselves by taking a daily multi-vitamin supplement.

Other immunity-boosting foods include:

- Almonds
- Blueberries
- Citrus fruits
- Garlic
- Green tea
- Green vegetables and dark green salad leaves
- Kale
- Kiwi

- Live yoghurt (check on the carton)
- Mushrooms
- Poultry
- Raspberries
- Red peppers
- Shellfish
- Spinach
- Sunflower seeds
- Turmeric

Antioxidants are important

Antioxidants are the 'good guys' and free radicals are the 'bad guys'. Antioxidants protect our cells, whilst free radicals are thought to play a role in causing heart disease, cancer and other diseases. Antioxidants are compounds in foods that scavenge and neutralise the free radicals in our body. Vitamins, minerals and other nutrients help to repair damaged cells and keep us healthy.

Fruit and vegetables that are brightly coloured are high in antioxidants – including beetroot, blueberries, broccoli, cabbage, carrots, kale, oranges, peppers, spinach, strawberries, tomatoes – but they are also found in non-brightly coloured foods such as ginger, garlic and onions.

Vitamins and minerals

Eating lots of fruit and vegetables is fabulous for our immune system as they are bursting with valuable antioxidants, minerals and vitamins, and particularly infection-fighting vitamin C. Fruit and vegetables are low in calories and high in vital fibre, which is crucial to our achieving a healthy gut. Whilst I have included unlimited salad and vegetables on this Eating Plan, fruit is restricted because of its high sugar content.

Here is a quick-reference list to help you to understand which vitamins and minerals are particularly important for our immune system, and where you can find them. If you recognise that there are some nutrients that you know are not included in your regular diet, then maybe consider taking a daily supplement.

Vitamin A – Helps our body's natural defence against illness and infection, boosting our immune system. Vitamin A can be found in:

- Oily fish
- Milk and yoghurt
- Liver
- Eggs
- Carrots
- Sweet potatoes
- Spinach
- Red peppers

Vitamin B Complex – This is a collection of B vitamins vital to our immune system and comprises eight different vitamins: B1 is thiamine, B2 is riboflavin, B3 is niacin, B5 is pantothenic acid, B6 is pyridoxine, B7 is biotin, B9 is folic acid and B12 is cobalamin. Each member of the vitamin B collection has an essential part to play in our body functioning and some of them are crucial to our immune system, particularly B6.

Vitamin B2 (riboflavin) helps break down fats and

medication. Vitamin B2 is found naturally in some foods and is often added to fortified foods. We can find it in eggs, liver and kidneys, lean meats, low-fat milk and green vegetables, including broccoli, spinach and asparagus.

Vitamin B6 (pyridoxine) is vital to keeping the immune system strong, making new red blood cells and transporting oxygen throughout the body. It is also responsible for producing white blood cells and T cells, which regulate our immune responses. Foods rich in B6 are chicken, tuna, leafy green vegetables and chickpeas.

Vitamin B9 (folate) is valuable during pregnancy as it can help reduce the risk of birth defects. This vitamin is found in broccoli, Brussels sprouts, leafy green vegetables, peas, kidney beans and chickpeas. The man-made version of folate is called folic acid and is often found in fortified breakfast cereals.

Vitamin B12 (cobalamin) improves nerve cells and can reduce the risk of developing anaemia and is mainly found in meat, offal, milk, fish and eggs. Vegetarians and vegans will find it harder to eat enough B12, though it is found in some fermented foods, such as tempeh, and, more commonly, in nori (a type of edible seaweed) and yeast extract, like Marmite.

As a general guide, you can find the B vitamins in:

- Milk
- Cheese
- Eggs
- Liver and kidney
- Meat, such as red meat and chicken
- Fish, such as tuna, mackerel and salmon

- Shellfish, such as oysters and clams
- Dark green vegetables, such as spinach and kale
- Wholegrain bread
- Seeds

Their very name – vitamin B complex – and their vital role in supporting our immune system suggests that taking a supplement may prove helpful in boosting your levels of immunity.

Vitamin C – This is a vital nutrient for health as it assists us in fighting infection. It helps form and maintain bones, skin and blood vessels and boosts our collagen levels. It occurs naturally in some foods, especially fruit and vegetables, but it cannot be stored in the body. It is for this reason that I have included within this Plan no restriction on the consumption of salad and vegetables at mealtimes. Some fruit is also included but because of its high sugar content, fruit is more restricted.

When we think of vitamin C we automatically think of citrus fruits like oranges, lemons and grapefruits as being very rich in this vitamin – which of course they are – but, interestingly, bright-coloured peppers are even more.

Fruit and vegetables high in vitamin C are:

- Kiwi fruit
- Strawberries
- Oranges
- Lemons
- Grapefruit
- Papayas
- Melon
- Tomatoes and tomato juice

- Kale
- Peas
- Broccoli
- Brussels sprouts
- Cauliflower
- Peppers – interestingly, red, yellow and orange peppers have more vitamin C than green ones
- Spinach
- Cabbage
- Leafy greens

Vitamin D – Our body creates vitamin D from direct sunlight on our skin when we are outdoors. This is why it is so important for us to go for our daily 30-minute walk. Vitamin D is important for our bones, teeth and muscles.

As well as from sunlight, we also get vitamin D from oily fish, such as salmon, mackerel, herring and sardines, and from red meat and eggs. For those following a plant-based diet, you will find that oat milk, soya milk or almond milk are usually fortified with vitamin D.

Vitamin E – This vitamin is another important vitamin for our immune system and it is found in vegetable oils such as wheatgerm, sunflower, safflower and almond oil. It will also be found in sunflower seeds, almonds and other nuts.

Vitamin F – This is a vitamin we don't hear so much about but it still has an important role to play in providing structure to our cells, it supports growth and development, and is involved in major bodily functions, such as blood pressure regulation and our immune response. Vitamin F can be found in egg yolks, chia seeds and almonds.

Vitamin K – This is a group of vitamins that our body needs for blood clotting and helping wounds to heal, which is why it falls into this 'immunity-boosting' category of helpful vitamins. There's also some evidence vitamin K helps keep bones healthy. We can find it in green leafy vegetables, like kale, spinach or broccoli. It can also be found in cereal grains – another reason to choose wholegrain varieties.

We only need 1 microgram a day of vitamin K per kilo of body weight and a microgram is 1,000 times smaller than a milligram – so it is a tiny amount. This is one vitamin that we should get sufficiently from our diet, so there is no need to take a supplement for this one.

Selenium – While we only need a very small amount, selenium plays a key role in our metabolism. We need it to protect our body from the damage caused by free radicals and from infection.

Whilst it's important that we have sufficient selenium to be healthy, eating a varied diet, including protein foods such as meat, fish, chicken, turkey, eggs, cottage cheese, beans, mushrooms, oats, sunflower seeds and some fortified cereals, should give us all we need. Some nuts, especially Brazil nuts, also contain selenium. There is no need to take a supplement of this mineral as it can be harmful to have too much.

Zinc – One very important immunity-fighting nutrient is zinc. Zinc is a mineral that plays a vital role as it is one of the most important components of the enzymes found in our immunity-fighting white blood cells, but zinc is absorbed better from protein sources rather than through supplements. The most natural source of zinc is from protein foods, such as red meat, fish, beans, chickpeas, lentils, tofu, nuts, chia seeds, ground linseed, hemp seeds, wholemeal bread, quinoa and milk.

The importance of fibre

Eating foods with high fibre content not only helps us stay healthy, it also supports us in controlling our weight. Foods high in fibre keep us feeling fuller for longer and allow our gut, our digestion and our bowels to work more efficiently, which, in turn, enhances our general health and well-being. Always look for high-fibre cereals and wholegrain bread, eat plenty of vegetables and salad and keep the skins on your new potatoes.

How Can We Boost Our Gut Health?

Gut health is emerging as a whole new area of fascinating science that is attracting a great deal of attention and discussion. We are now learning that gut health is not only important to our general well-being, but is also vital in boosting our immune system, helping to prevent illness and disease, particularly as we get older.

The inhabitants of our gut, the microbes (a microbe is a microscopic organism that is found within our body), were until recently almost impossible to study, but then came the genetic revolution and we were able to track fragments of bacteria that live in our gut by detecting their DNA. The result is that now scientists know which type of bacteria should be in our gut and that has helped us understand what we ought to be eating. This allows us to create the very best way to stay healthy and this, in turn, helps us to boost our immune system.

Our body contains trillions of microbes and many of them are good for us, and some not so good. The biggest population of these microbes is found in our gut and what we eat can change them, which can dramatically affect our health – positively and negatively. Microbes play a critical role in our digestion, our immune function and in the regulation of our weight. By eating a healthy diet, we create more good bacteria and less bad bacteria within our gut. Here are three good reasons to have a healthy gut:

- **It can help you lose weight.** Those microbes can decide how much energy our body extracts from food. There are certain good microbes that, if we have enough of them, are associated with low levels of obesity, while one particular microbe is linked to following regular periods of fasting, say from 7 p.m. to 7 a.m. the next day, which has been proven to help in the control of weight.
- **It can boost our immune system.** Improving the balance of 'good vs bad' bacteria in our gut can effectively reduce the number of coughs and colds we get and has even been linked to reducing our risk of contracting flu, which in later years presents a real threat. For this to

happen, we need more of the friendly, good bacteria and less of the unfriendly, bad bacteria. Good bacteria are a valuable asset to our gut as they greatly enhance the activity of the immune system by crowding out and killing the bad bacteria, thus giving the immune system a real 'boost'.

- **It can enhance our mental health.** There is significant research currently being undertaken in this area. There is some evidence that the bacteria in our gut can also affect our brain. Apparently, parts of our food that cannot be digested are converted into chemicals that can enhance our mood and hopefully reduce our chances of becoming depressed. This is a very exciting area of research.

What can we do to boost our immune system?

Our first step is to eat the foods that the friendly, good bacteria thrive on. These foods are called prebiotics. Then we need to add more of those living microbes to ensure that they stay 'top dogs' in our gut, fighting and winning the battle against the unfriendly, bad bacteria. These are called probiotics

A **prebiotic** is a special type of plant fibre that your body cannot digest, but which encourages the growth of valuable good bacteria. The 'good gut bacteria' then turn that prebiotic fibre into valuable chemicals that have a powerful anti-inflammatory effect. You can think of them as being like a form of fertiliser, boosting the growth of good bacteria. Some good examples are:

- Asparagus
- Garlic
- Grains
- Leeks
- Legumes, such as pulses, peas and beans
- Onions
- Seeds

Probiotics offer helpful bacteria found in foods that contain live cultures. The ones we are most familiar with are live yoghurt and kefir. They contain live organisms of specific strains of bacteria that add to the population of friendly, good bacteria in the gut. They have the ability to attack and destroy disease-causing bacteria. In fact, it is the opposite of what antibiotics do, which, whilst fighting infection, have the ability to destroy *all* forms of bacteria, so weakening your immune system. If you are forced to take antibiotics it is important to take probiotics on a daily basis to protect your levels of good bacteria. Examples of probiotics are:

- Apple cider vinegar
- Kimchi
- Live kefir
- Live yoghurt
- Miso soup
- Sauerkraut
- Sour cream

Branded probiotics are readily available in supermarkets, such as Yakult and Actimel, and provide a convenient and helpful solution to providing valuable friendly, good bacteria to our daily diet. Alternatively, prebiotic and probiotic supplements are widely available from health stores or online.

Why exercise is good for your gut

It makes a lot of sense that any regular and varied movement that an exercise programme provides will help the function of the gut. For food to move freely through the digestive system and be usefully absorbed, it not only needs the types of foods mentioned in this book, but also we need plenty of physical activity. By following a regular, full-body exercise programme, which this book recommends, alongside improving your eating habits, you will complete the necessary elements to achieve your most precious goal – the very best of health!

3. The Enemies of Our Immune System

So far, we have discussed in some detail the benefits of losing a few pounds and increasing the nutrients that boost our immune system, enabling us to have our best chance of fighting infections and viruses should they come our way. But eating well and shedding weight is only half the story.

There is little point in making all this effort if we then abuse our body by smoking, eating in excess and devouring unhealthy food or by drinking too much alcohol.

These are some of the things that work against us and that the body has to *fight against* for us to stay healthy. Here they are:

Smoking

We all know that smoking is harmful to our health and a potential killer. If you are currently a smoker, by quitting now you will be doing the very best thing you can do to boost your immunity and give yourself a chance to live longer.

Alcohol

Alcohol is a mixture of good and bad. It is a relaxant and it has been acknowledged by the medical profession that having a glass of wine can be beneficial in helping to relieve stress, thus helping to reduce the risk of heart disease. The problem is that few of us stop at a single glass. It is, however, a mild form of poison and the body works very hard to get rid of it. Since alcohol is a toxin, and the body has no useful reason to store it, the body works really hard to prioritise the elimination of it at the cost of processing the health-giving food that we eat. Obviously, this is bad news for our immune system. Consequently, whilst following this plan, try to avoid alcohol – or at least keep consumption to a minimum.

Caffeine

Caffeine is a stimulant, which can increase our heart rate and our blood pressure, so it can impact our overall health. It may also hinder our sleep pattern among many other side-effects. Whilst following this plan, like alcohol, please try to keep your caffeine consumption to a minimum. Regular tea contains half the caffeine of coffee, and by taking your tea weak, you can reduce the caffeine significantly more. Green tea and fruit teas contain no caffeine. You don't have to cut out caffeine, just think about cutting it back a little.

Sugar

Sugar contains empty calories, which means it offers no nutrients. All it does is give us energy. If we are eating fruit and vegetables, we will be getting plenty of natural sugar anyway. The problem we have with sugar is that we often eat it combined with saturated fat in desserts, confectionery, pies, cakes and biscuits. These calorie-dense products easily cause unwanted weight gain, but the effect on our health can be far more damaging than just a few extra pounds. When we become overweight or obese, we become at significantly greater risk of heart disease, Type 2 diabetes and some cancers. If we are trying really hard to build our immunity and become healthier, cutting right back on sugar is a great place to start, and that means cutting back on sugary drinks and snacks too.

Butter and margarine

Saturated fats such as butter and margarine are not good for our heart health. All fat contains twice as many calories as protein and carbohydrate, so it makes sense to cut right back if we are trying to lose weight. When eating bread and toast, try spreading toppings straight onto the bread to save unnecessary saturated fat. Be mindful of low-fat substitute products available in supermarkets and look at the ingredients. Some products are created with a vast selection of artificial components, which offer very little goodness.

Unsaturated fats such as olive, rapeseed, flaxseed and many other plant-based oils are healthy, but because they are around 100 per cent fat, we should keep consumption to a minimum when trying to lose weight. Using an oil spray when cooking offers an effective low-calorie alternative.

Cakes and biscuits

Cakes and biscuits should only be eaten as an occasional treat. If eaten regularly they will undoubtedly add a few inches to your waistline and increase your chances of suffering from heart problems, Type 2 diabetes, increase your risk of suffering a stroke and some cancers. Anyone who makes their own cakes will know how much fat and sugar goes into making most of them. If we add some jam, cream or buttercream as a filling or topping, they take the calorie count even higher.

When it comes to biscuits, there is an easy test to determine the fat content, whether sweet or savoury. The more fat they contain, the easier they are to break. The problem with biscuits is that we rarely stop at one and they come in packets, which makes nibbling very easy. If you have them in the house, they will tempt you, so leave them off your shopping list.

If you want to lose weight, stay healthy and keep your immune system fighting fit, try to say 'no' to cakes and biscuits.

Pastries and pies

Pastry is made with fat – usually saturated fat – and the lighter the pastry, the more fat it contains. Savoury pastry also usually contains a lot of salt, so if you want to get and stay healthy, plus boost your immune system, please say 'no' to pastries and pies too.

Meat products (e.g. salami, pâté, scotch eggs, sausage rolls, sausages and bacon)

Meat 'products' and processed meat are loosely described as meat-based foods manufactured using pork, poultry, lamb or beef to create a savoury product. This process often involves using fragments of meat combined with fat and, to make them more palatable, lots of salt. Meat products are considered to be significantly less healthy than pure meat or poultry, normally have a high saturated fat and salt content and are usually high in calories.

Junk food and some takeaways

As the name suggests, burgers, deep-fried fast-food and high-fat takeaways provide limited nutritional value. With a high fat and salt content and minimal valuable nutrients, they work against our efforts to become healthier and fitter. In addition, because of the low fibre content, junk food has poor satiety value. In other words, it doesn't keep you feeling full for long enough and very soon you find yourself feeling hungry again. If you want to be healthy, give junk food and unhealthy takeaways a miss.

Deep-fried food

Chips, crisps and savoury snacks that are deep-fried are adding loads of unnecessary calories and lots of unhealthy salt to our body. The oil they are cooked in is 100 per cent fat and, to make deep-fried food palatable, it is served with lots of salt, which is bad news for our heart health.

Whilst having a very occasional bag of fish and chips wouldn't be the end of the world, try to make it a rare treat rather than a regular habit.

Avoid snacking

I personally believe that snacking is probably the biggest reason why the majority of our nation is getting fatter.

We snack between meals for two reasons – out of habit or because we haven't eaten sufficiently at mealtimes. If we eat nutritious food, it will give us valuable nutrients to boost our immune system, satisfy our appetite and keep us feeling fuller for longer. This means that our body won't crave food halfway through the morning or afternoon. This is such an important fact to take on board.

As was mentioned by my trialists, they 'welcomed' the fact that this eating plan had 'rules' – we *can* eat as much salad and vegetables as we want at mealtimes, and eat three meals a day, but we should *avoid* eating unhealthy foods and stop the snacking habit. The message is crystal clear:

To enjoy maximum benefit from this 28-day plan, we are asking you to stop snacking.

4. The 28-Day Immunity-Boosting Weight-loss Plan

The focus on staying healthy has never been greater than it is now. But, just imagine how wonderful you will feel if you follow our 28-day Immunity-Boosting Weight-loss Plan AND lose 7–14lbs!

Research has proven that when dieters lose weight fast, their motivation to continue is much greater. With this in mind, I have designed the optimum weight-loss plan that will keep you well nourished, your appetite satisfied and your immune system boosted. The hope is that after the 28 days you will feel so much better that you will want to carry on eating healthily and being more active into the long term – just as my trialists did.

What You Need to Do

Daily allowance

- Milk allowance: 425ml (¾ pint) semi-skimmed milk (dairy or plant-based).
- Eat three meals a day: Keep to the Immunity-Boosting Weight-loss Plan for 28 days, following the breakfast, lunch and dinner options.

- Dessert: 100g live natural yoghurt or live kefir OR
  1 probiotic drink, plus one of the following fruit:
  1 apple with skin
  1 fun-sized mini banana (or ½ full-sized one)
  60g blueberries
  150g fresh fruit salad
  12 seedless grapes
  2 kiwi fruit
  200g melon
  1 large peach or nectarine
  1 pear with skin
  100g fresh pineapple
  200g raspberries
  2 satsumas or similar
  150g strawberries

Alternatively, if you choose not to have live yoghurt, kefir or a probiotic drink, you can select any two portions from the fruits listed above.

Diet Notes

All meals are interchangeable

This is a 'pick 'n' mix' eating plan, so you can select the breakfast or lunch you like and eat it every day if you wish. In recipes, substitute meat, poultry and fish with vegetarian alternatives as desired. If you don't have all the ingredients of a recipe, adapt it to suit what you do have.

Desserts

The dessert option may be taken after your main meal of the day or at any time to suit your desire or convenience. You may also, if you wish, break it up into two healthy mini-meals if needed, e.g. 11 a.m.: 75g strawberries with 50g live yoghurt and later, the remaining 75g strawberries with the remaining 50g of live yoghurt.

Vegetarian/vegan options

There is a vegetarian or vegan alternative for all dinner options in the Plan.

Recipes

Most recipes are for two people, but if you wish to serve more, increase the ingredients accordingly. Recipes that are for four/six portions are suitable for freezing.

Keep hydrated

Drink as much water as you wish. Tea is unlimited, made with milk from the daily allowance or, better still, drink green tea if you like it. Please keep coffee to a minimum. Low-calorie drinks are unlimited, including low-sugar squash.

Alcohol

Alcohol is a toxin that the body has to fight to eliminate from our system. The last thing we need at this time is to use up our body's valuable resources in fighting a toxin we don't need to invite in. So, during this time, keep alcohol to an absolute minimum.

Yoghurt and kefir with live cultures

These offer us a rich source of probiotics. These are vital to our gut health, which helps fight infections. They also strengthen our digestive system and our gut flora by providing 'good' bacteria to help populate the gut. There are various brands of yoghurt available in supermarkets with live cultures, including Yeo Valley, Rachel's and Onken. In this eating plan I have used live natural yoghurt or kefir, to which you can add fresh fruit.

Frying with rapeseed oil spray

This is ideal to add flavour to stir-fries, omelettes and other recipes when using a non-stick pan, and it will save you lots of unnecessary calories. It is available at your local supermarket.

Gravy

Make gravy with the water in which you have cooked your vegetables as this contains more nutrients. Bisto gravy powder is low in fat and easy to use. Mix with a little cold water first, then add to the hot vegetable water and stir continually until boiling.

Vegetable stock cubes

These add significant flavour when added to the cooking water used to prepare vegetables, potatoes, pasta and rice.

Bread

Wholegrain bread is made with unrefined flour, so provides more fibre. Wholemeal, wholewheat and wholegrain bread are basically different terms for the same thing and all are wholegrain.

Alternatives to fat

In sandwiches, try spreading your wholemeal bread with low-fat dressings in preference to saturated fats. Products such as Branston Pickle, low-fat salad dressing, extra-light soft cheese, HP Sauce, fruity sauce, tomato ketchup, Marmite, mustard and horseradish sauce are great alternatives, which can be spread straight onto the bread.

Record Your Progress (see page 286)

Weigh yourself once a week on the same scales and at the same time and write it down.
Measure yourself around the narrowest measurement around your waist every week and write it down.

The Eating Plan

Day 1

BREAKFAST: 2 x normal Weetabix and 1 teaspoon demerara sugar (or 14 x Fruit & Nut Weetabix Minis) with milk from allowance, plus a piece of fruit (vegetarian)

LUNCH: 300ml **Mixed Vegetable Soup** (see page 70), plus 1 slice of wholemeal bread (no butter) (vegan)

DINNER: **Spaghetti Bolognese** (see page 90) (with vegetarian option)

OR **Prawn Curry** (see page 118)

Day 2

BREAKFAST: 150g live yoghurt mixed with 150g raspberries or strawberries (vegetarian)

LUNCH: 2 slices of wholemeal toast topped with 200g baked beans (vegan)

DINNER: **Chicken and Pepper Stir-Fry** (see page 105) with rice

OR **Sweet Potato, Green Bean and Cauliflower Curry** (see page 148) (vegan)

Day 3

BREAKFAST: 1 small slice of wholemeal toast spread with Marmite with 1 egg, poached or boiled, plus an orange (vegetarian)

LUNCH: *Crunchy Salad* – chopped pepper, cucumber, celery, mushrooms, grated carrot, sliced red onion, cherry tomatoes and bean sprouts mixed with 1 tablespoon cooked basmati rice and 1 tablespoon of peas and sweetcorn. Dress with a low-fat dressing or soy sauce and serve with 2 tablespoons cold baked beans (vegetarian)

DINNER: 200g cod steak, steamed or microwaved, served with 100g new potatoes, in their skins, plus unlimited fresh vegetables

OR **Spicy Beef with Beans and Tomatoes** (see page 100) served with a baked sweet potato in its jacket and unlimited vegetables or salad

OR **Marjoram-Stuffed Peppers** (see page 155) served with 100g new potatoes, in their skins, plus unlimited fresh vegetables (vegan)

Day 4

BREAKFAST: 50g Fruit 'n Fibre with milk from allowance and 1 teaspoon demerara sugar (vegetarian)

LUNCH: 1 sliced banana, 200g strawberries or raspberries, plus a sliced pear served with 3 tablespoons live yoghurt (vegetarian)

OR **Fresh Tomato and Basil Soup** (see page 75), plus 1 slice of wholegrain bread (vegan)

DINNER: **Chilli con Carne** (see page 85) (with vegetarian option)

OR **Vegetable Chilli** (see page 133) (vegan)

Day 5

BREAKFAST: 4 pieces of fresh fruit (excluding bananas) (vegan)

LUNCH: ¼ portion of **Chilli Beans** (see page 137), plus 1 slice of wholemeal bread (vegan)

DINNER: 2-egg omelette with mushrooms fried in a non-stick pan sprayed with rapeseed oil, plus unlimited salad (vegetarian)

OR **Chicken Casserole** (see page 112) served with 100g new potatoes, in their skins, plus unlimited other vegetables

Day 6

BREAKFAST: 50g Special K cereal and 1 teaspoon brown sugar with milk from allowance (vegetarian)

LUNCH: Spread 2 slices of wholemeal bread with horseradish sauce or low-fat salad dressing and make into a jumbo sandwich with 30g wafer-thin beef, chicken, ham, tofu or chickpeas, plus unlimited salad vegetables (with vegetarian option)

DINNER: 150g roast chicken breast (no skin) served with 1 small **Dry-roasted Sweet Potato** (see page 164), plus unlimited vegetables and low-fat gravy

OR **Parsnip Cakes with Red Pepper Relish** (see page 157) (vegan)

Day 7

BREAKFAST: 30g All-bran and 1 teaspoon demerara sugar with milk from allowance, plus a boiled egg (vegetarian)

LUNCH: *Salmon Wraps* – spread a tortilla wrap with 1 teaspoon Thai sweet chilli dipping sauce, then fill with 25g smoked or cooked salmon or mackerel, chopped salad leaves, peppers, cucumber, celery and cherry tomatoes. Wrap up as a parcel, tucking in the edges as you roll it up. Cut in half horizontally to make two wraps

For a vegetarian alternative, use quinoa in place of fish (vegan)

DINNER: *Chicken Pasta* – Place 100g chopped chicken breast (no skin), ½ chopped onion, 1 crushed garlic clove and some freshly ground black pepper in a large non-stick pan sprayed with rapeseed oil and toss the chicken in the pan until it changes colour. Add a sliced green pepper, a tin of chopped tomatoes, ½ finely chopped small fresh chilli (optional) and a dash of Worcestershire sauce and allow to simmer for

5 minutes. Serve with 45g pasta (dry weight) cooked in boiling water with a vegetable stock cube

OR **Broccoli and Pepper Stir-Fry with Noodles** (see page 128) (vegan)

Day 8

BREAKFAST: 1 small glass (125ml) fresh orange juice with 1 slice of wholemeal bread spread with Marmite, plus a boiled egg (vegetarian)

LUNCH: *Mixed Bean Salad* – mix together 100g drained tinned chickpeas, 100g red kidney beans, rinsed, and 25g sweetcorn kernels. Add 2 sliced spring onions or ½ finely chopped red onion, 3 halved cherry tomatoes, chopped celery and cucumber and ½ finely chopped pepper. Mix together well. Stir in some chopped fresh coriander and basil and toss in balsamic vinegar or a low-fat dressing of your choice. Add freshly ground black pepper to taste (vegan)

Note: You can use the remaining beans from the **Chilli Beans** recipe (see page 137)

DINNER: *Oven-baked Salmon* – place 1 x 100g salmon steak in an ovenproof dish and top with 1 teaspoon Thai sweet chilli dipping sauce and the juice of ½ lemon or lime. Bake in a preheated 200°C/400°F/gas 6 oven for 8 to 10 minutes, or until just cooked. Do not overcook. Serve with 100g new potatoes, in their skins, plus unlimited vegetables or salad

OR **Cottage Pie with Leek and Potato** (see page 96) served with unlimited vegetables

OR **Roast Vegetable and Lentil Dhal** (see page 145) (vegan)

Day 9

BREAKFAST: 2 scrambled eggs with unlimited tinned tomatoes and mushrooms fried in a non-stick pan sprayed with rapeseed oil (vegetarian)

LUNCH: Halve 1 medium wholemeal roll, spread with horseradish sauce, mustard or low-fat salad dressing and top each half with 30g wafer-thin beef, chicken, ham, tofu or chickpeas, some sliced tomatoes and cucumber (with vegetarian option)

DINNER: **Tomato, Basil and Lemon Penne** (see page 154) (vegan)

OR **Lamb and Pearl Barley Casserole** (see page 98) served with unlimited green vegetables

Day 10

BREAKFAST: The night before, take 20g uncooked porridge oats, 10 sultanas, 1 teaspoon sunflower seeds and a handful of chopped almonds and mix with 2 tablespoons live yoghurt and 1 teaspoon runny honey and place in the fridge. In the morning, add a little milk from allowance to soften the mixture, if desired, before eating (vegetarian)

LUNCH: 300ml **Carrot and Coriander Soup** (see page 68) (vegan)

DINNER: 1 well-grilled lamb chop served with 100g new potatoes, in their skins, plus unlimited vegetables and low-fat gravy

OR **Chilli Pinto Bean Burritos** (see page 159) (vegan)

Day 11

BREAKFAST: 40g muesli (any brand) and 1 teaspoon demerara sugar with milk from allowance (vegetarian)

LUNCH: 150g chopped cooked chicken served with chopped peppers, cucumber, celery, cherry tomatoes, mushrooms and grated carrot and beetroot, plus bean sprouts. Dress with soy sauce

For a vegetarian alternative, use quinoa in place of chicken (vegan)

OR **Rich Red Lentil Soup** (see page 79) (vegetarian)

DINNER: *Fish Pie* – place 50g each of salmon, cod and prawns in a small ovenproof dish. Cover with ⅓ tin of condensed cream of mushroom soup* and top with mashed potato (made by boiling 115g floury potatoes and mashing with milk from allowance. Season well). Place the pie on a baking tray and bake in a preheated 200°C/400°F/gas 6 oven for 30 minutes or until the potato is brown on top. Serve with unlimited vegetables

*Use the remaining mushroom soup for tomorrow's lunch

OR **Beef and Pepper Kebabs with Teriyaki Sauce** (see page 103)

OR **Rich Mushroom Tagliatelle** (see page 152) (vegetarian)

Day 12

BREAKFAST: 40g porridge oats soaked in 250ml boiling water in a pan overnight. Reheat and serve with milk from allowance and 2 teaspoons runny honey (vegetarian)

LUNCH: Heat ⅔ tin of condensed cream of mushroom soup, reconstituted as described on the tin, and serve with 1 slice of wholemeal toast (vegetarian)

DINNER: *Baked Liver and Onions* – place 150g calves' liver in an ovenproof dish with a finely sliced onion. Cover with a lid or foil and bake in a preheated 180°C/350°F/gas 4 oven for 15 minutes until lightly cooked. Make gravy with vegetable stock and a little Bisto gravy powder. When boiling, add to the liver and onion and cook for a further 5 minutes. Serve with 100g new potatoes, in their skins, plus unlimited vegetables

OR **Salmon Pasta Salad** (see page 168) served with salad leaves

OR 250ml any **Soup** (see pages 68–82), plus 1 large baked sweet potato with **Stir-Fried Mushrooms and Peppers** (see page 130) (vegan)

Day 13

BREAKFAST: 2 large bananas (vegan)

LUNCH: 4 rye crackers or 1 slice of wholemeal bread, spread with Philadelphia Light Soft Cheese with Garlic and Herbs, plus cherry tomatoes and cucumber and a small salad (vegetarian)

OR **Roasted Garlic and Green Pea Soup** (see page 81), plus 1 slice of wholegrain bread (vegetarian)

DINNER: *Super Booster Salad Bowl* – use a low-fat dressing of your choice between each layer as you place the following alternately into a serving bowl: dark salad leaves, 100g shredded smoked or cooked salmon or prawns, sliced peppers, radishes, tomatoes, cucumber, celery, courgettes and mushrooms and cubes of melon and mango

OR **Roasted Vegetable Curry** (see page 146) (vegan)

Day 14

BREAKFAST: 50g Fruit 'n Fibre with milk from allowance and 1 teaspoon brown sugar, plus 100g raspberries or strawberries (vegetarian)

LUNCH: **Italian Vegetable Soup** (see page 77) (vegan)

DINNER: **Thai Sweet Chilli Chicken** (see page 108) served with 55g basmati rice (dry weight) cooked in boiling water with a vegetable stock cube

OR **Quorn Thai Red Curry** (see page 150) (vegan)

Day 15

BREAKFAST: 200g live yoghurt mixed with 1 teaspoon honey and 10 chopped almonds (vegetarian)

LUNCH: 4 Ryvitas or similar high-fibre crispbreads, spread with Marmite and topped with 2 sliced hard-boiled eggs and a salad (vegetarian)

OR **Stuffed Mushrooms** (see page 163) served with a small salad (vegetarian)

DINNER: **Cottage Pie** (see page 88) (with vegetarian option) served with unlimited vegetables

OR **Spicy Lemon Chicken** (see page 110) served with new potatoes, in their skins, and unlimited vegetables

Day 16

BREAKFAST: 2 boiled eggs (vegetarian)

LUNCH: 120g cooked chicken breast mixed with a *Waldorf salad* – 1 chopped apple, 2 chopped sticks of celery, 10 sultanas, 4 chopped walnut halves and shredded salad leaves mixed with 2 teaspoons low-fat dressing and 2 teaspoons live yoghurt. Toss well, then mix in the chicken

DINNER: *Chilli Prawn Stir-fry with Asparagus* – place ½ chopped red onion and 1 crushed clove of garlic in a large non-stick pan sprayed with rapeseed oil and cook until soft. Add 50g asparagus and 100g raw peeled prawns and cook for 2 to 3 minutes until the prawns change colour. Pour in a small sachet of chilli stir-fry sauce and stir well to coat the prawns and asparagus. Heat through and serve with unlimited salad

OR **Stir-Fried Vegetables with Ginger and Sesame Sauce** (see page 126) (vegan)

Day 17

BREAKFAST: 1 slice of wholemeal toast topped with 200g baked beans (vegan)

LUNCH: 1 large **Dry Roasted Sweet Potato** topped with 50g smoked mackerel, salmon or pilchards mixed with low-fat salad cream and served with unlimited salad

DINNER: **Beef and Ale Stew** (see page 87) served with 100g mashed potato and unlimited vegetables

OR **Chickpea and Root Vegetable Stew with Couscous** (see page 131) served with unlimited vegetables (vegan)

Day 18

BREAKFAST: 2 rashers of well-grilled lean back bacon served with unlimited grilled tomatoes and mushrooms

LUNCH: 120g tin of sardines in tomato sauce served on 2 slices of wholemeal toast

DINNER: **Ginger Beef Stir-Fry** (see page 83)

OR **Citrus and Ginger Pappardelle Stir-Fry** (see page 123) (vegan)

Day 19

BREAKFAST: 1 slice of wholemeal toast topped with 1 scrambled egg and a large grilled tomato (vegetarian)

LUNCH: 1 wholemeal pitta bread opened up and spread inside with Thai sweet chilli dipping sauce and filled with 50g salmon (or vegetarian alternative), shredded leaves and mixed salad vegetables (with vegetarian option)

DINNER: 125g roast chicken and 1 **Dry-Roasted Sweet Potato** (see page 164) served with unlimited vegetables

OR **Blackeye Beans with Ginger and Soy** (see page 138) (vegan)

Day 20

BREAKFAST: 150g strawberries served with 100g live yoghurt (vegetarian)

LUNCH: 2-egg omelette served with unlimited mushrooms fried in a non-stick pan sprayed with rapeseed oil, plus unlimited salad (vegetarian)

DINNER: 120g grilled beef steak served with 150g new potatoes, in their skins, plus unlimited vegetables or salad

OR **Aubergine Tagine with Couscous** (see page 140) (vegan)

Day 21

BREAKFAST: 1 large sliced banana mixed with 100g live yoghurt and 100g raspberries (vegetarian)

LUNCH: 1 large baked sweet potato, topped with **Home-Made Coleslaw** (see page 165) and served with unlimited salad (vegetarian)

DINNER: **Horseradish Fish Pie** (see page 116)

OR **Tofu Indonesian-Style** (see page 161) (vegan)

Day 22

BREAKFAST: 4 dried prunes, soaked in hot black tea overnight, served with 100g live yoghurt (vegetarian)

LUNCH: **Sweet Potato and Leek Soup** (see page 73) (vegetarian)

DINNER: **Tandoori Salmon with Spicy Noodles** (see page 122)

OR **Teriyaki Tempeh with Rice and Broccoli** (see page 160) (vegan)

Day 23

BREAKFAST: 2 fresh peaches or nectarines served with 100g live yoghurt (vegetarian)

LUNCH: 300ml **Spicy Butternut Squash Soup** (see page 71), plus 1 slice of wholemeal bread or toast (vegan)

DINNER: 1 large **Dry-Roasted Sweet Potato** (see page 164), topped with 75g tuna mixed with a low-fat salad dressing or 200g baked beans, served with salad (with vegan option)

OR **Austrian-Style Beef Goulash** (see page 94) served with unlimited green vegetables

Day 24

BREAKFAST: 1 slice of well-grilled back bacon served with ½ slice of wholemeal toast and an egg and 100g mushrooms fried in a non-stick pan sprayed with rapeseed oil

LUNCH: Mixed salad of leaves, watercress, cherry tomatoes, cucumber, onion, red and green peppers, mushrooms, bean sprouts and grated carrot, dressed with a low-fat salad dressing, soy sauce or balsamic vinegar. Serve with 100g wafer-thin ham, chicken or beef or salmon, mackerel or sardines in tomato sauce

OR **Home-Made Coleslaw** (see page 165) with 100g cold baked beans (vegetarian)

DINNER: **Chicken Korma** (see page 107) served with salad

OR **Baked Aubergine with Chickpeas, Bulgur and Feta-Style Cheese** (see page 141) served with unlimited salad (vegan)

Day 25

BREAKFAST: 100g blueberries served with 150g live yoghurt (vegetarian)

LUNCH: *Garlic Mushrooms with Bacon* – Cook unlimited button mushrooms in a non-stick pan sprayed with rapeseed oil. Add 2 crushed cloves of garlic together with 2 chopped rashers of bacon and cook until crispy. Serve with unlimited vegetables or salad (excluding potatoes)

DINNER: **Roast Vegetable and Chickpea Pasta** (see page 153) (vegan)

OR **Beef Curry** (see page 101) served with rice

Day 26

BREAKFAST: 1 slice of wholemeal toast topped with a 400g tin of plum tomatoes that have been boiled down to reduce the liquid (vegan)

LUNCH: 1 chicken breast served with unlimited salad and a low-fat dressing

For a vegetarian alternative, use 100g quinoa in place of the chicken with 1 tablespoon seeds of your choice (vegetarian)

OR **French Onion Soup** (see page 74), plus 1 slice of wholegrain bread (vegan)

DINNER: **Asian Salmon Steaks with Stir-Fried Veg** (see page 115)

OR **Quorn, Pepper and Mushrooms Stir-Fry** (see page 125) (vegan)

Day 27

BREAKFAST: 2 Shredded Wheat and 2 teaspoons brown sugar with milk from allowance, plus a piece of fruit (vegetarian)

LUNCH: **Smoked Mackerel Pâté** (see page 114) served with 4 rye crispbreads and a small salad

DINNER: **Sardine and Tomato Tagliatelle** (see page 121)

OR **Spicy Chickpea Casserole** (see page 135) (vegetarian)

Day 28

BREAKFAST: 150g live yoghurt mixed with 100g mixed fruit salad (vegetarian)

LUNCH: 2 slices of wholemeal bread spread with low-fat cream cheese, topped with 50g smoked salmon and cucumber slices, plus a small salad

DINNER: **Beef and Quorn Burgers** (see page 92)

OR **Arrabbiata Prawns with Rice** (see page 120)

OR **Lentil and Roast Vegetable Loaf** (see page 143) (vegan) served with **Marinated Roast Vegetables** (see page 166) (vegan)

5. Immunity-Boosting Recipes

SOUPS

Carrot and Coriander Soup (vegan)

Serves 4
Per serving: 140 calories, 0.9g fat
Prep 10 minutes
Cook 30 minutes

This flavoursome soup really benefits from being made the day before you eat it and stored in the fridge or freezer. Choose young, crisp carrots as these tend to be sweet and you may find they don't need peeling.

- 3 onions, chopped
- 1 clove of garlic, crushed
- rapeseed oil spray
- 450g carrots, peeled and diced
- 600ml vegetable stock (use 2 stock cubes)
- 1 tablespoon ground coriander
- freshly ground black pepper
- 2 tablespoons chopped fresh coriander, to garnish

Place the onion and garlic in a large non-stick pan sprayed with rapeseed oil and cook until soft.

Add the carrot, stock and ground coriander and bring to the boil. Reduce the heat and simmer for 20 minutes.

Allow to cool slightly, then pour into a blender or food processor and purée until smooth.

Return the soup to the pan to warm up, add the coriander and season to taste with the pepper.

If using a soup maker, add the fresh coriander when pulsing for the second time.

Mixed Vegetable Soup (vegan)

Serves 4–6
Per serving: depends on vegetables used
Prep 10 minutes
Cook 30 minutes

This is a great soup to make when you have surplus vegetables that need using up. This soup freezes well too.

- 3 onions, chopped
- rapeseed oil spray
- use one each of any root vegetables to hand (potato, sweet potato, carrot, parsnip, swede), diced
- add any available cabbage, celery or leeks, trimmed and chopped
- 500ml vegetable stock (use 2 stock cubes)
- 2 tablespoons chopped fresh coriander
- freshly ground black pepper

Place the onion in a large non-stick pan sprayed with rapeseed oil and cook until soft.

Add the vegetables and stock and bring to the boil. Reduce the heat and simmer for 20 minutes.

Allow to cool slightly, then pour into a blender or food processor and purée until smooth.

Add the coriander, season to taste with the pepper and whiz again. If it's too thick, don't worry, just add a little more water or stock when heating up to serve.

If using a soup maker, add the fresh coriander when pulsing for the second time.

Spicy Butternut Squash Soup (vegan)

Serves 4
Per serving: 67 calories, 1.2% fat
Prep 20 minutes
Cook 30 minutes

A delicious soup that can be made in advance and freezes well.

- 1 small butternut squash
- rapeseed oil spray
- 115g young, crisp carrots, sliced
- 2 onions, chopped
- 2 cloves of garlic, crushed
- 2 sticks of celery, chopped
- 1–2 teaspoons medium curry powder (e.g. tandoori spice mix)
- 1.2 litres vegetable stock
- freshly ground black pepper

Cut the squash in half lengthways. Remove the seeds with a spoon and discard. Using a sharp vegetable knife, peel away the thick skin and cut the flesh into chunks.

Preheat a large non-stick saucepan and spray with rapeseed oil.

Place the squash and the other vegetables in the hot pan and fry for 4 to 5 minutes until they soften and start to colour.

Add the curry powder and cook out for 1 minute, keeping the mixture moving to prevent it catching on the bottom of the pan. Gradually pour in the vegetable stock, stirring continuously, then bring to the boil.

Reduce the heat and simmer until the vegetables are tender.

Allow to cool slightly, then pour into a blender or food processor and purée until smooth.

Return the soup to the pan to warm up, adjusting the consistency with a little extra stock if needed. Taste and season with pepper.

If using a soup maker, in this recipe it is important to fry the vegetables first before placing in the soup maker to cook.

Sweet Potato and Leek Soup (vegetarian)

Serves 2
Per serving: 244 calories, 1% fat
Prep 10 minutes
Cook 40 minutes

- 2 large leeks, chopped
- rapeseed oil spray
- 300g sweet potato, peeled and diced
- 2 cloves of garlic, crushed
- 1 litre vegetable stock
- 300ml semi-skimmed milk
- optional: chopped fresh chives, to garnish

Place the leek in a large non-stick pan sprayed with rapeseed oil and cook for 1 to 2 minutes until soft.

Add the potato, garlic and stock and bring to the boil. Reduce the heat and simmer until the potato is soft.

Allow to cool slightly, then pour into a blender or food processor and purée until smooth.

Return the soup to the pan to warm up, add the milk and bring back up to near boiling. Sprinkle with chives and serve.

French Onion Soup (vegan)

Serves 8
Per serving: 95 calories, 1.2g fat (excluding accompaniments)
Prep 10 minutes
Cook 25 minutes

This tasty low-fat recipe is suitable for freezing and is a great alternative to the usual high-fat version.

- 675g large onions, sliced
- 1.2 litres vegetable stock (use stock cubes if preferred)
- 2 cloves of garlic, crushed
- 1 tablespoon chopped fresh thyme
- 2 tablespoons plain flour
- freshly ground black pepper
- 2 tablespoons chopped fresh parsley, to garnish

Place the onions in a large pan with a little of the vegetable stock.

Sweat the onions until soft. Add the garlic and thyme. Sprinkle the flour over and mix well. Season with black pepper and cook for a moment or two to 'cook out' the flour, stirring continuously.

Gradually add the remaining stock, stirring well, bring to the boil and simmer for 10 minutes.

Just before serving, sprinkle with the parsley and serve with wholegrain bread.

Fresh Tomato and Basil Soup (vegan)

Serves 4
Per serving: 115 calories, 1.1g fat (excluding accompaniments)
Prep 10 minutes
Cook 30 minutes

This soup will keep in a refrigerator for three days and is suitable for freezing.

- 3 onions, finely chopped
- rapeseed oil spray
- 1kg fresh ripe tomatoes
- 2 cloves of garlic, crushed
- 2 tablespoons tomato purée
- 300ml cold water
- 2 vegetable stock cubes
- handful of fresh basil leaves
- freshly ground black pepper

Place the onion in a large non-stick frying pan or saucepan sprayed with rapeseed oil and cook until soft, then set aside.

Meanwhile, place the tomatoes in a bowl, pour over boiling water and leave for 3 minutes. Prepare another bowl of ice-cold water with ice cubes. Remove the tomatoes from the boiling water with a slotted spoon, place them straight into the ice-cold water and leave for 3 minutes to allow the skins to split.

Peel the tomatoes – the skins should come away easily – and put the skins in a sieve placed over a bowl or saucepan to collect any juices.

Cut the peeled tomatoes into four and remove the seeds and the core. Place the deseeded tomatoes in the pan with the onion and place the seeds, core and any juices into the sieve to collect any juices that pass through. Using the back of a wooden spoon, press the discarded core, seeds and skin to extract as much juice as possible, then add the drained juice to the pan.

Add the garlic, tomato purée, cold water and crumbled stock cubes to the pan with the onion and tomato. Bring to the boil, then add freshly ground black pepper and simmer for 15 to 20 minutes.

Allow to cool slightly, then pour into a blender or food processor and purée until smooth. Add the basil leaves and purée again for 30 seconds.

Return the soup to the pan to warm up, season to taste and serve hot with a slice of wholegrain bread.

If using a soup maker, fry the onion, then place all the ingredients, except the basil, but including the deseeded tomatoes, into the soup maker and cook for 20 minutes on High. When cooked, pulse for 30 seconds. Add the basil and pulse for another 30 seconds.

Italian Vegetable Soup (vegan)

Serves 2
Per serving: 252 calories, 3.9g fat
Prep 10 minutes
Cook 30 minutes

This soup will provide a substantial lunch.

- 2 carrots, thinly sliced
- 2 leeks, thinly sliced
- 1 red pepper, deseeded and cut into 5mm dice
- 1–2 sticks of celery, thinly sliced
- 1 onion, thinly sliced
- a few dark Savoy cabbage leaves, finely shredded
- 1 x 400g tin of chopped tomatoes
- 2 cloves of garlic, crushed
- 1 bay leaf
- 1.2 litres vegetable stock including a vegetable stock cube
- 50g very small pasta shapes or dried spaghetti, broken into 1cm pieces (see note)
- 1 tablespoon chopped fresh oregano
- freshly ground black pepper

Place all the vegetables and the chopped tomatoes in a large saucepan.

Add the garlic, bay leaf and vegetable stock with the stock cube. Bring to the boil and simmer for 30 minutes until the vegetables are tender.

Fifteen minutes before the end of the cooking time, add the pasta and oregano. When cooked, remove the bay leaf and season to taste with freshly ground black pepper.

Note: The easiest way to break the spaghetti is to wrap it in a tea towel and break it over the edge of the work top, adding a little pressure. Unfold the tea towel and add the broken spaghetti strands into the soup.

Rich Red Lentil Soup (vegetarian)

Serves 4
Per serving: 254 calories, 1.3g fat
Prep 20 minutes
Cook 25 minutes

This is a really easy and tasty cook-in-the-pot soup. You can make it in advance and keep it in the refrigerator for 5 days and it is also suitable for freezing.

- rapeseed oil spray
- 1 onion, chopped
- 1 clove of garlic, crushed
- 2 sticks of celery, chopped
- 2 carrots, chopped
- optional: 2 teaspoons chopped fresh thyme
- 1 teaspoon ground cumin
- 175g dried red lentils
- 1 litre vegetable stock (use 2 stock cubes if preferred)
- 1 x 400g tin of chopped tomatoes
- 2 tablespoons live natural yoghurt
- freshly ground black pepper
- optional: 1 tablespoon chopped fresh parsley, to garnish

Spray a large non-stick saucepan with rapeseed oil spray and fry the onion until soft.

Add the remaining ingredients, except the yoghurt, and bring to the boil. Reduce the heat and simmer gently for 20 minutes until the lentils are soft.

Allow to cool slightly, then blend with a stick blender or purée in small batches in a food processor. Thin the soup down with a little extra vegetable stock or water if needed.

Return the soup to the pan to warm up. Just before serving, remove from the heat, stir in the yoghurt and season to taste with black pepper.

Serve into warm bowls and garnish with chopped parsley.

Roasted Garlic and Green Pea Soup (vegetarian)

Serves 4
Per serving: 85 calories, 1.7g fat
Prep 10 minutes
Cook 1 hour

This delicious vegetarian soup is suitable for freezing.

- 1 whole head of garlic (see note)
- 450g frozen petits pois
- 1 onion, finely chopped
- 600ml vegetable stock (use stock cubes if preferred)
- 8 fresh mint leaves
- freshly ground black pepper
- 1 tablespoon live natural yoghurt, to serve

Preheat the oven to 200°C/400°F/gas 6.

First, roast the garlic. Remove the outer skin from the garlic bulb or slice the top off. Place on a square of foil and wrap the foil around to form a parcel. Place in the oven for 45 minutes until soft.

Place the peas and chopped onion in a large saucepan and barely cover with the vegetable stock. Boil for 15 minutes.

Pour into a blender or food processor and purée until smooth.

Squeeze out the garlic purée from the roasted bulb and add to the blender or food processor with the mint and the vegetable stock and blend again until smooth.

Return the soup to the pan to warm up. Season to taste with freshly ground black pepper and just before serving, stir in the yoghurt.

Note: As the garlic needs to be roasted for approximately 45 minutes before you make the soup, you can roast it beforehand when using the oven for something else, then wrap it in foil and store in your refrigerator for up to a week. Roasting the garlic gives it a gentler flavour.

MEAT

Ginger Beef Stir-Fry

Serves 2
Per serving: 397 calories, 2% fat
Prep 20 minutes
Cook 15 minutes

- 200g thin beef steak, sliced
- 110g basmati rice
- 1 vegetable stock cube
- ½ red onion, sliced
- rapeseed oil spray
- ½ red pepper, deseeded and thinly sliced
- 1 stick of celery, thinly sliced
- 200g tinned bean sprouts, drained

for the marinade

- 1 tablespoon dark soy sauce
- 1 tablespoon sherry
- ½ teaspoon sugar
- 2 teaspoons very finely chopped fresh ginger
- 1 tablespoon light soy sauce

Place the beef in a bowl. Mix together all the marinade ingredients and pour over the beef. Leave to marinate for 30 minutes.

Five minutes before you start stir-frying, cook the rice in boiling water with a vegetable stock cube according to the packet instructions. When cooked, drain well and keep hot.

Place the onion in a large non-stick pan sprayed with rapeseed oil and cook until soft. Add the pepper and celery and cook for 1 to 2 minutes, then add the beef and toss together until the beef is almost cooked. Finally, add the drained bean sprouts and heat through. For a stronger flavour add the marinade to the pan two minutes before serving.

Serve the stir-fry with the rice.

Chilli Con Carne (with vegetarian option)

Serves 6
Per serving: 246 calories, 2.5% fat
Prep 10 minutes
Cook 40 minutes

Make in advance and freeze.

- 1 large onion, diced
- 2 cloves of garlic, crushed
- rapeseed oil spray
- 500g extra-lean minced beef (or vegetarian alternative)
- 2 teaspoons chopped fresh thyme
- 1 beef stock cube (or vegetable stock cube)
- 1 red pepper, deseeded and thinly sliced
- 1 small fresh red chilli, deseeded and sliced (or use a few dried chilli flakes)
- 400g tin of chopped tomatoes
- 400g tin of kidney beans, rinsed
- 300g tomato passata
- 1 tablespoon tomato purée
- freshly ground black pepper
- 55g basmati rice per person

Place the onion and garlic in a large non-stick pan sprayed with rapeseed oil and cook until soft. Add the mince and thyme and continue cooking to brown the mince.

Sprinkle the stock cube over the mince, then add the

red pepper, chilli, tomatoes, kidney beans, tomato passata and tomato purée. Simmer gently for 25 minutes until the sauce has thickened and the beef is tender. Add freshly ground black pepper to taste.

Page 103: Beef and Pepper Kebabs with Teriyaki Sauce

Page 114: Smoked Mackerel Pâté

Page 159: Chilli
Pinto Bean Burritos

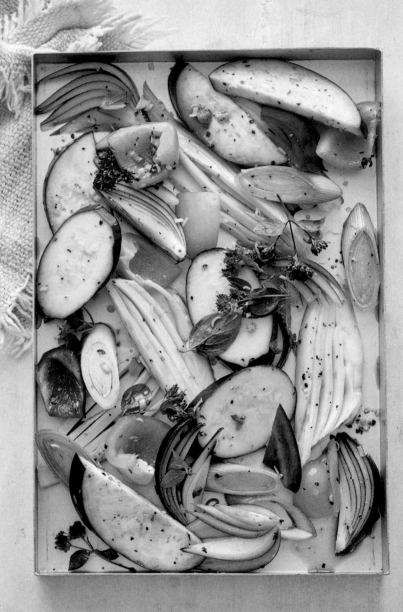

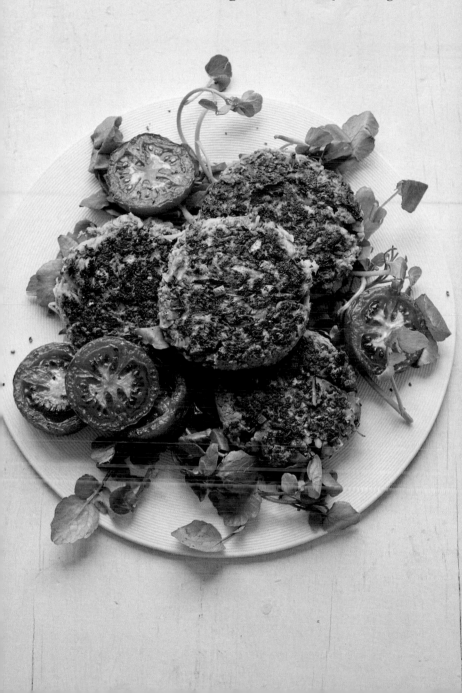

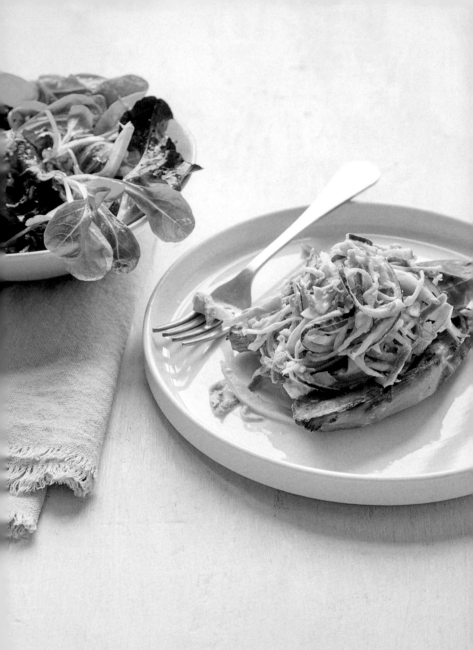

Page 164—5: Dry-Roasted Sweet Potatoes topped with Home-Made Coleslaw

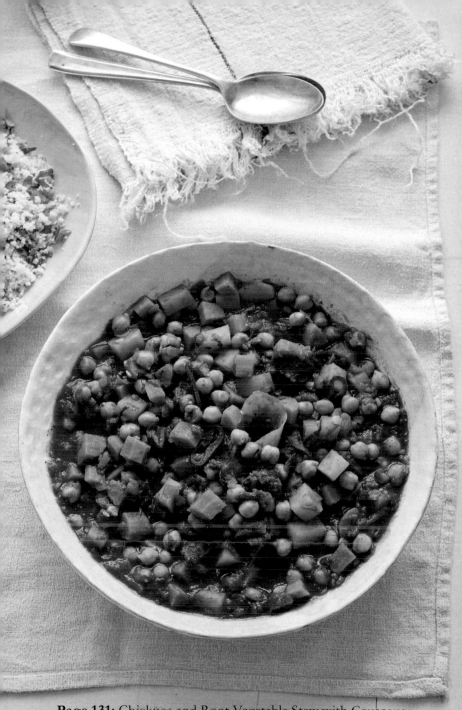

Page 131: Chickpea and Root Vegetable Stew with Couscous

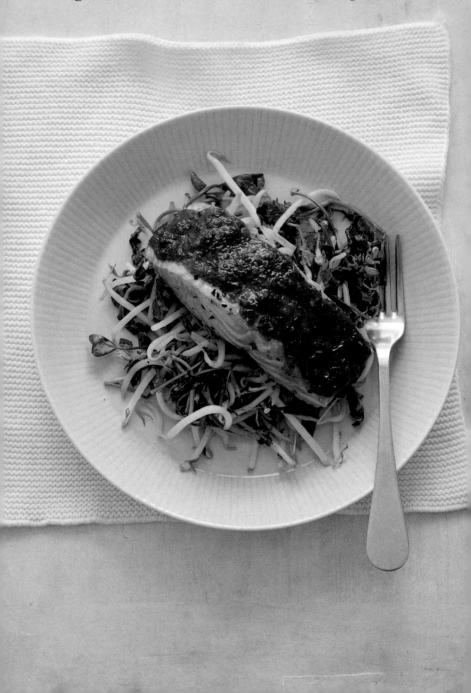

Beef and Ale Stew

Serves 2
Per serving: 256 calories, 8.7g fat
Prep 10 minutes
Cook 1 hour 15 minutes

- 1 red onion, diced
- 1 clove of garlic, crushed
- rapeseed oil spray
- 200g lean diced beef
- 1 stick of celery, chopped
- 10g sun-dried tomatoes, chopped
- 250ml ale or stout
- 250ml beef stock
- 1 tablespoon gravy granules
- 150g small button mushrooms
- 2 teaspoons mixed herbs (parsley, thyme, chives)
- freshly ground black pepper

Place the onion and garlic in a large non-stick pan sprayed with rapeseed oil and cook until they start to brown.

Add the beef, season with black pepper and continue cooking to seal the meat.

Add the celery, tomatoes and beer or stout and bring to the boil. Stir in the beef stock and gravy granules, add the mushrooms and herbs, then cover and simmer gently for 1 hour until the meat is tender.

When the meat is tender, adjust the consistency of the sauce by adding more gravy granules or water and serve straight away with unlimited green vegetables.

Cottage Pie (with vegetarian option)

Serves 2
Per serving: 400 calories, 2.8% fat (excluding
    accompaniments)
Prep 5 minutes
Cook 40 minutes

- 2 large sweet potatoes, peeled and cut into small chunks
- 1 vegetable stock cube
- 1 onion, finely chopped
- 200g extra-lean minced beef (or vegetarian alternative)
- 1 large carrot, peeled and grated
- 1 tablespoon meat or vegetable gravy granules
- 1 beef stock cube (or vegetable stock cube)
- a little milk from daily allowance
- freshly ground black pepper

Cook the potatoes in a pan of boiling water containing the vegetable stock cube until tender. Drain, reserving the cooking water for the gravy later.

Meanwhile, preheat a non-stick wok or frying pan. Add the onion and mince and dry-fry until it changes colour. Add the carrot and mix in well, then turn off the heat.

Preheat the oven to 200°C/400°F/gas 6.

Start to make the gravy by mixing the gravy granules with a little cold water in a jug.

Heat 300ml of the reserved potato cooking water and the crumbled beef stock cube in a pan and stir well.

When hot, slowly add the mixed gravy granules, stirring continuously to prevent it from going lumpy. When boiling, add some gravy into the mince mixture, then pour into a small/medium-sized pie dish, reserving some gravy for serving later.

Mash the potatoes, adding a little milk from your allowance and some pepper until smooth.

Carefully pile the mashed potato on top of the mince, making sure the potato is sealed to the edges to prevent the gravy bubbling out during cooking.

Place the cottage pie on a baking tray in the oven and cook for 20 minutes.

Serve with unlimited vegetables and the remaining gravy.

Spaghetti Bolognese (with vegetarian option)

Serves 4
Per serving: 398 calories, 8.9g fat
Prep 15 minutes
Cook 40 minutes

- 300g lean minced beef (or vegetarian alternative)
- 2 cloves of garlic, crushed
- 1 large onion, finely diced
- 2 carrots, grated
- 1 beef or vegetable stock cube
- 2 x 400g tins of chopped tomatoes
- 2 tablespoons tomato purée
- 1 tablespoon chopped fresh mixed herbs (oregano, marjoram, basil)
- 220g spaghetti
- 1 vegetable stock cube
- optional: chopped fresh basil
- freshly ground black pepper

Dry-fry the minced beef in a non-stick pan until it starts to change colour. Add the garlic and onion and continue cooking for a further 2 to 3 minutes, stirring well.

Add the carrot and crumble the stock cube over the top. Add the chopped tomatoes, tomato purée and mixed herbs and mix well to allow the stock cube to dissolve. Reduce the heat to a gentle simmer, season, cover with a lid and continue to cook for 30 minutes until the sauce thickens.

Cook the pasta in a pan of boiling water containing the vegetable stock cube, according to the packet instructions. Drain.

Just before serving, add the chopped fresh basil, if using, to the sauce.

Arrange the spaghetti on warmed serving plates and pour the sauce on top.

Note: Bolognese sauce can be frozen.

Beef and Quorn Burgers

Serves 4
Per serving: 182 calories, 4.6% fat (excluding
 accompaniments)
Prep 10 minutes
Chill 10 minutes
Cook 25 minutes

Choose mustard or horseradish to flavour these simple
burgers.

- 300g extra-lean minced beef
- 100g Quorn mince
- 2 cloves of garlic, crushed
- 1 red onion, finely chopped
- 1 medium courgette, grated
- 1 teaspoon grain mustard or horseradish
  sauce
- 1 teaspoon vegetable stock powder
- freshly ground black pepper

Squeeze the grated courgette to remove any excess
liquid, then combine all the ingredients together in a bowl
and season with black pepper.

Divide the mixture into four portions and then, using
your hands, mould each portion into a ball. Place them on
a board and use a palette knife to shape each ball into a
flat round shape. Chill for 10 minutes.

Preheat a non-stick pan then, when the burgers are
chilled, dry-fry them for about 10 minutes, or until cooked
as you like, turning halfway through.

Serve with new potatoes, in their skins, and 1 grilled tomato per person, plus unlimited additional vegetables.

Note: These can be frozen if the minced beef is fresh and has not been previously frozen.

Austrian-Style Beef Goulash

Serves 4
Per serving: 429 calories,15.7g fat (excluding accompaniments)
Prep 15 minutes
Cook 2 hours 30 minutes

This goulash is suitable for freezing.

- rapeseed oil spray
- 2 large onions, sliced
- 675g lean stewing steak, cut into cubes
- 2 carrots, diced
- 2 sticks of celery, chopped
- 1 tablespoon plain flour
- 1½ tablespoons mild paprika
- 600ml beef stock (use stock cubes if preferred)
- 1 tablespoon chopped fresh thyme
- 2 bay leaves
- 2 tablespoons tomato purée
- freshly ground black pepper
- optional: chopped fresh mint and parsley, to garnish

Preheat the oven to 180°C/350°F/gas 4.

Heat a non-stick pan or casserole dish sprayed with rapeseed oil until hot and fry the onion until soft. Add the beef, a little at a time to maintain the heat in the pan, to sear the sides of the chunks. Season well with freshly ground black pepper.

Add the carrot and celery and cook for a further minute. Reduce the heat, sprinkle with the flour and paprika and stir to 'cook out' the flour for another minute. Then gradually add the stock, stirring continually to avoid lumps forming. Add the thyme, bay leaves and tomato purée.

Cover the casserole and cook in the oven for approximately 2 hours or until the meat is tender.

When ready to serve, sprinkle over the chopped mint and parsley.

Serve with new potatoes, in their skins, plus unlimited green vegetables.

Cottage Pie with Leek and Potato

Serves 2
Per serving: 327 calories, 6.2g fat (excluding accompaniments)
Prep 10 minutes
Cook 50 minutes

for the topping

- 340g potatoes, peeled and chopped
- 2 leeks, sliced
- 2 tablespoons milk

for the mince

- 225g lean minced beef
- 1 onion, chopped
- 2 carrots, coarsely grated
- 1 tablespoon plain flour
- 150ml beef stock (use a stock cube if preferred)
- 2 teaspoons tomato purée
- 2 teaspoons mixed dried herbs
- freshly ground black pepper

Preheat the oven to 190°C/375°F/gas 5.

Cook the potatoes in a pan of boiling water until softened, adding the leeks 5 minutes before the end of the cooking time.

Heat a non-stick frying pan, add the mince and dry-fry for 3 to 4 minutes.

Add the onion and carrot to the pan and stir in the flour. Gradually add the stock, tomato purée and herbs. Bring to the boil and stir until thickened. Season with black pepper and transfer to a small/medium-sized oven-proof dish.

Drain the potatoes and leeks and mash with a little milk. Season to taste. Carefully arrange the mash on top of the mince mixture, using the back of a fork to smooth it over.

Bake in the oven for 25 minutes until crisp and golden on top. Serve with unlimited vegetables.

Lamb and Pearl Barley Casserole

Serves 2

Per serving: 402 calories, 10.5g fat (excluding accompaniments)

Prep 15 minutes, plus soaking

Cook 1 hour 45 minutes

It is very important that the lentils and beans are soaked overnight for this tasty casserole as they cannot be cooked directly from their dried state.

- rapeseed oil spray
- 1 onion, diced
- 1 clove of garlic, crushed
- 225g lean diced lamb
- 2 carrots, diced
- 1 small turnip, peeled and diced
- 225g small new potatoes
- 1 stick of celery, chopped
- 500ml beef, lamb or vegetable stock (use a stock cube if preferred)
- bouquet garni
- 25g green lentils, soaked overnight
- 12g haricot beans, soaked overnight
- 12g pearl barley
- freshly ground black pepper
- optional: 1 tablespoon chopped fresh parsley

Heat a non-stick pan and spray with rapeseed oil. Add the onion and garlic and fry for 2 to 3 minutes until soft.

Add the lamb, seasoning well with black pepper, and continue to cook over a high heat until well sealed.

Transfer to a large casserole dish and add the remaining vegetables, the stock and the bouquet garni.

Rinse the soaked lentils, beans and the pearl barley well and add to the casserole.

Cover and simmer gently for 1 hour or until the meat is tender, topping up with additional stock if required.

Remove the bouquet garni and, just before serving, sprinkle with fresh parsley.

Serve with unlimited green vegetables.

Spicy Beef with Beans and Tomatoes

Serves 4
Per serving: 212 calories, 6.4g fat (excluding accompaniments)
Prep 20 minutes
Cook 30 minutes

This beef chilli is suitable for freezing.

- rapeseed oil spray
- 1 red onion, finely chopped
- 225g lean minced beef
- 2 cloves of garlic, crushed
- 1 red pepper, deseeded and finely sliced
- 1 x 400g tin of chopped tomatoes
- 1 fresh red chilli, deseeded and finely chopped
- 1 x 400g tin of red kidney beans, rinsed
- 600ml beef stock (use a stock cube if preferred)
- freshly ground black pepper

Preheat a non-stick frying pan and spray with rapeseed oil. Add the onion to the pan and cook until soft.

Add the minced beef to the pan and fry until browned. Add the crushed garlic and red pepper and cook for 2 to 3 minutes more.

Transfer the mixture to a saucepan and add the tomatoes, chilli, kidney beans and beef stock, bringing the pot to a gentle simmer for 20 minutes to allow the sauce to thicken.

Season to taste with black pepper.

Serve with a baked sweet potato in its jacket and unlimited vegetables or salad.

Beef Curry

Serves 2
Per serving: 415 calories, 6.4g fat
Prep 5 minutes
Cook 15 minutes

This beef curry is ideal when you want a quick meal, though leaving it to simmer for longer will enhance the flavour and it is even better prepared the day before and left overnight before reheating.

- 110g basmati rice
- 1 vegetable stock cube
- rapeseed oil spray
- 1 onion, finely chopped
- 1 clove of garlic, crushed
- 225g lean beef rump, cut into thin strips
- 1 tablespoon Madras curry powder or paste
- 1 courgette, diced
- 1 x 400g tin of chopped tomatoes
- freshly ground black pepper
- 1 tablespoon chopped fresh coriander, to garnish
- 1 tablespoon live natural yoghurt, to serve

Cook the rice in boiling water with a vegetable stock cube according to the packet instructions. When cooked, drain well and keep hot.

Meanwhile, heat a large non-stick frying pan and spray with rapeseed oil. Fry the onion for 2 to 3 minutes until soft. Add the garlic and the beef and cook for a further 2 to 3 minutes until the beef is browned.

Add the curry powder or paste and cook for a further minute, stirring well. Add the courgette and tomatoes and season well with black pepper. Simmer for 3 to 4 minutes until the sauce thickens.

Remove the beef curry from the heat, stir in the fresh coriander and yoghurt and serve immediately with the boiled rice.

Beef and Pepper Kebabs with Teriyaki Sauce

Serves 2
Per serving: 361 calories, 4.9g fat
Prep 5 minutes
Cook 25 minutes

This dish also works well with chicken or lamb and is great served with a fresh salad.

for the kebabs

- 350g extra-thin beef steaks, cut into thin strips
- 1 green and 1 orange or red pepper, deseeded and cut into squares
- 110g basmati rice
- 1 vegetable stock cube

for the sauce

- 3 tablespoons soy sauce
- 3 tablespoons dry sherry
- 1 clove of garlic, crushed
- 1 small teaspoon ground ginger
- 1 teaspoon dark brown sugar

Thread the beef strips, concertina style, onto four skewers, placing a square each of green and orange/red pepper between each strip.

Cook the rice in boiling water with a vegetable stock cube according to the packet instructions. When cooked, drain well and keep hot.

To make the sauce, place all the ingredients in a small pan and heat gently until simmering, stirring occasionally.

Allow the sauce to simmer on a very low heat while you cook the rice.

Preheat the grill.

Place the skewers on a grill pan and brush a little sauce over the meat and peppers. Cook under the preheated grill for 5 to 8 minutes, turning regularly and basting occasionally with more of the sauce.

Arrange the skewers on plates and pour the remaining sauce over the meat. Serve with the rice.

POULTRY

Chicken and Pepper Stir-Fry

Serves 1

Per serving: 432 calories, 3.4g fat or 276 calories, 2.4g fat
(excluding rice)

Prep 10 minutes

Cook 15 minutes

- 55g basmati rice
- 1 vegetable stock cube
- 1 clove of garlic, crushed
- 1 chicken breast, chopped
- rapeseed oil spray
- ½ red onion, roughly chopped
- ½ red and ½ green pepper, deseeded and chopped
  into bite-sized squares
- 2 sticks of celery, chopped
- 4 button mushrooms, halved
- a little grated fresh ginger
- 1 teaspoon honey
- 2 tablespoons soy sauce, plus more to serve
- 1 tablespoon chilli and garlic sauce
- optional: fresh coriander
- freshly ground black pepper

Cook the rice in boiling water with the vegetable stock
cube according to the packet instructions. When cooked,
drain well and keep hot.

Meanwhile, place the garlic, chicken and some pepper

in a large non-stick pan sprayed with rapeseed oil and fry until almost cooked.

Add the red onion, peppers, celery and mushrooms and toss with the chicken. Do not overcook the vegetables.

Add the grated ginger with the honey, soy and chilli and garlic sauces and the fresh coriander, if using, and mix well.

Serve immediately, with soy sauce if required.

Chicken Korma

Serves 2

Per serving: 233 calories, 1.5% fat (excluding
  accompaniments)

Prep 10 minutes

Cook 20 minutes

- 1 small onion, chopped
- rapeseed oil spray
- 1 clove of garlic, crushed
- 225g lean diced chicken
- 1 tablespoon mild curry powder
- ½ tablespoon plain flour
- ½ teaspoon ground cinnamon
- 150ml chicken stock
- freshly ground black pepper
- 150g low-fat natural yoghurt, to serve
- 1 tablespoon chopped fresh coriander, to garnish

Place the onion in a large non-stick pan sprayed with
rapeseed oil and cook until soft. Add the garlic and the
chicken and cook for 2 to 3 minutes until the chicken
changes colour.

Sprinkle the curry powder and flour over the chicken.
Toss the chicken so that it is completely covered, then add
the cinnamon and cook for 1 minute.

Gradually add the stock, stirring well, and season to
taste with the pepper. Simmer gently for 10 minutes until
the sauce thickens.

Remove the pan from the heat, stir in the yoghurt and
coriander and serve immediately with salad (no rice).

Thai Sweet Chilli Chicken

Serves 1
Per serving: 408 calories, 0.6% fat
Prep 10 minutes
Cook 20 minutes

- 100g skinless chicken breast
- ½ red pepper, deseeded and finely sliced
- 2 spring onions, finely chopped
- 2 plum tomatoes, skinned, deseeded and diced
- 3 tablespoons Thai sweet chilli dipping sauce
- 2 cloves of garlic, crushed
- a pinch of ground cumin
- a pinch of ground coriander
- 1 teaspoon cornflour
- 75ml pineapple juice
- 55g basmati rice
- 1 vegetable stock cube
- freshly ground black pepper
- chopped fresh coriander, to garnish

Preheat the oven to 190°C/375°F/gas 5.

Place the chicken in a small ovenproof dish (with lid) and season on both sides with the pepper.

Place the red pepper, spring onion and tomato in a bowl. Add the dipping sauce, garlic, cumin and coriander and combine well.

Dissolve the cornflour in the pineapple juice and pour over the vegetables and spices. Mix well and season with pepper. Pour the vegetables, with the juice, over the chicken and bake for 20 minutes.

While the chicken is in the oven, cook the rice in boiling water with a vegetable stock cube according to the packet instructions. When cooked, drain well and keep hot.

Serve the chicken with the rice and sprinkled with fresh coriander.

Spicy Lemon Chicken

Serves 2
Per serving: 186 calories, 2.5g fat (excluding accompaniments)
Prep 10 minutes, plus 1 hour marinating
Cook 15 minutes

Lemongrass is available fresh or dried, but using fresh lemongrass will enhance the finished dish.

- 2 skinless chicken breasts, cut into chunks
- zest and juice of 1 lemon
- 1 tablespoon light soy sauce
- ½ teaspoon ground coriander
- 75g tomato passata
- ½ small fresh red chilli, deseeded and finely sliced
- 1 teaspoon finely chopped lemongrass
- 1 clove of garlic, crushed
- rapeseed oil spray
- 2 teaspoons chopped fresh coriander
- freshly ground black pepper

Place the chicken in a shallow dish and season with black pepper.

Combine all the remaining ingredients, except the oil spray and fresh coriander, and pour over the chicken. Cover and leave to marinate for at least 1 hour, mixing occasionally.

Strain away the marinade from the chicken and reserve. Preheat a non-stick wok or frying pan and spray with rapeseed oil. Fry the chicken quickly over a high heat for 5 to 6 minutes, turning it regularly, to seal it on all sides.

Now add the reserved marinade and continue to cook for a further 10 minutes to allow the sauce to simmer gently and thicken. Stir in the fresh coriander and serve with new potatoes, in their skins, plus unlimited vegetables.

Chicken Casserole

Serves 2
Per serving: 235 calories, 8.6g fat (excluding accompaniments)
Prep 10 minutes
Cook 55 minutes

This all-in-one casserole combines chicken and vegetables in a rich tomato sauce. Fresh herbs give the sauce a real taste of Provence.

- rapeseed oil spray
- 1 onion, finely chopped
- 2 large skinless chicken breasts
- 1 clove of garlic, crushed
- 75ml chicken stock (use a stock cube if preferred)
- ½ tablespoon plain flour
- optional: 2 tablespoons red wine
- 1 x 400g tin of chopped tomatoes
- 2 teaspoons chopped fresh mixed herbs
- 75g baby chestnut mushrooms
- 1 small swede, peeled and diced
- freshly ground black pepper
- optional: 1 tablespoon chopped fresh parsley

Preheat the oven to 190°C/375°F/gas 5.

Heat a large non-stick frying pan sprayed with rapeseed oil and fry the onion until soft.

Season the chicken on both sides with black pepper and add to the pan, lightly browning on each side. Remove and place in an ovenproof dish.

Add the garlic and 2 tablespoons of the stock to the

onion and stir in the flour. 'Cook out' for 1 minute, then add the remaining stock, wine (if using) and the tomatoes. Stir in the mixed herbs, mushrooms and swede and bring to the boil. Pour over the chicken and cover with aluminium foil.

Bake in the centre of the oven for 30 to 35 minutes.

Just before serving, sprinkle with the chopped fresh parsley and serve with new potatoes, in their skins, plus unlimited other vegetables.

FISH AND SEAFOOD
Smoked Mackerel Pâté

Serves 6

Per serving: 165 calories, 19.5% fat (excluding accompaniments)

Prep 10 minutes

The pâté makes a great filling for jacket potatoes.

- 250g smoked mackerel fillets
- 1 tablespoon horseradish sauce
- 2 teaspoons grain mustard
- 1 tablespoon 2%-fat Greek yoghurt
- 2 spring onions, finely chopped
- optional: 2 teaspoons lime juice
- freshly ground black pepper

Using a fork, break the fish away from the skin and place into a bowl. Add the horseradish sauce, mustard, yoghurt and spring onions, mix well and season with plenty of pepper.

Press the mixture into six ramekins or small serving pots and chill until required.

Serve with rye crispbread.

Note: Once made, this pâté will keep for up to 5 days in the fridge. It is also suitable for freezing, providing the mackerel has not previously been frozen.

Asian Salmon Steaks with Stir-Fried Veg

Serves 2
Per serving: 414 calories, 4.8% fat
Prep 15 minutes
Cook 15 minutes

- 2 salmon steaks (150g each)
- rapeseed oil spray
- 2 teaspoons finely grated lemon zest
- 2 teaspoons chilli and garlic sauce
- 1 tablespoon Thai sweet chilli dipping sauce
- 310g pack of bean sprouts
- 100g watercress
- 150ml pineapple juice
- freshly ground black pepper

Preheat the oven to 200°C/400°F/gas 6.

Place the salmon steaks on a non-stick baking tray sprayed with rapeseed oil and season on both sides with the pepper.

In a small bowl, mix together the lemon zest, chilli and garlic sauce and chilli sauce and then drizzle it over the steaks.

Bake the steaks in the oven for 8 to 10 minutes until just cooked.

Meanwhile, heat a non-stick wok or frying pan sprayed with a little rapeseed oil and just before the salmon is cooked, stir-fry the bean sprouts and watercress until just wilted, then add the pineapple juice.

Transfer the wilted vegetables to two serving plates and top with the salmon steaks. Serve hot or cold.

Horseradish Fish Pie

Serves 2
Per serving: 130 calories, 1.1% fat (excluding
   accompaniments)
Prep 20 minutes
Cook 45 minutes

- 125g floury potatoes, peeled
- 100g sweet potatoes, peeled
- 1 vegetable stock cube
- 200ml semi-skimmed milk, plus extra for mashing
  the potatoes
- 1 tablespoon chopped fresh parsley
- 185g mixed chunky boneless fish (e.g. cod, hake,
  haddock)
- 1 tablespoon cornflour
- 1 small teaspoon vegetable stock powder
- 2 teaspoons horseradish sauce
- ½ teaspoon Dijon mustard
- rapeseed oil spray
- freshly ground black pepper

Preheat the oven to 200°C/400°F/gas 6.

Cook the floury and sweet potatoes in a pan of boiling
water with the vegetable stock cube, then drain and mash,
adding a little cold milk and the chopped parsley.

Meanwhile, cut the fish into bite-sized pieces and place
in the bottom of a small/medium ovenproof dish.

Mix the cornflour with a little cold milk to a paste, then
heat the remaining milk in a saucepan. When hot, whisk
in the cornflour paste to thicken the sauce. Stir in the

stock powder, horseradish and mustard and season with black pepper. Pour this over the fish and level the top with the back of a spoon. Cover with the mashed potatoes and lightly spray with rapeseed oil spray.

Place on a baking tray and bake in the oven for 20 to 25 minutes until golden brown. Serve hot with unlimited vegetables.

Prawn Curry

Serves 2
Per serving: 345 calories, 2.2g fat
Prep 25 minutes
Cook 25 minutes

- 110g basmati rice
- 1 vegetable stock cube
- 300ml fish or vegetable stock
- rapeseed oil spray
- 1 red onion, finely chopped
- 1 tablespoon tomato purée
- 2 teaspoons tamarind paste
- 2 kaffir lime leaves
- 225g raw peeled prawns
- 1 tablespoon chopped fresh coriander

for the paste

- 2 cloves of garlic
- 2 teaspoons ground coriander
- ¼ teaspoon ground turmeric
- ¼ teaspoon fenugreek seeds
- 2 small fresh chillies
- 2 cardamom pods, crushed and seeds removed

Cook the rice in boiling water with a vegetable stock cube according to the packet instructions. When cooked, drain well and keep hot.

Make the paste by grinding all the paste ingredients in a food processor or blender. Scrape the paste into a bowl,

Page 81: Roasted Garlic and Green Pea Soup

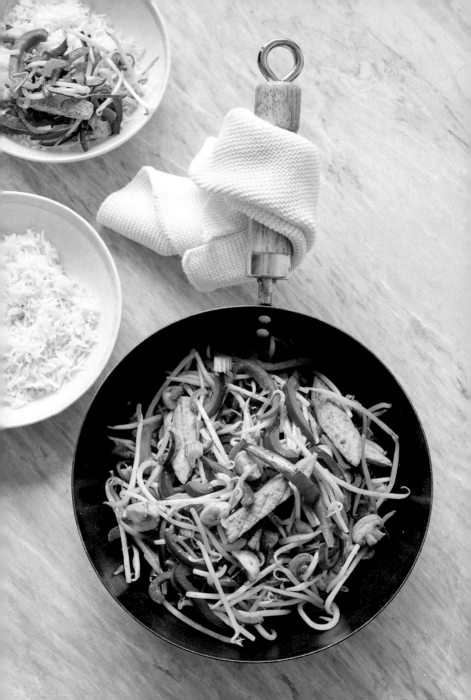

Page 125: Quorn, Pepper and Mushrooms Stir-Fry

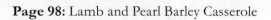

Page 98: Lamb and Pearl Barley Casserole

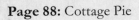
Page 88: Cottage Pie

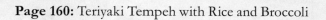

Page 160: Teriyaki Tempeh with Rice and Broccoli

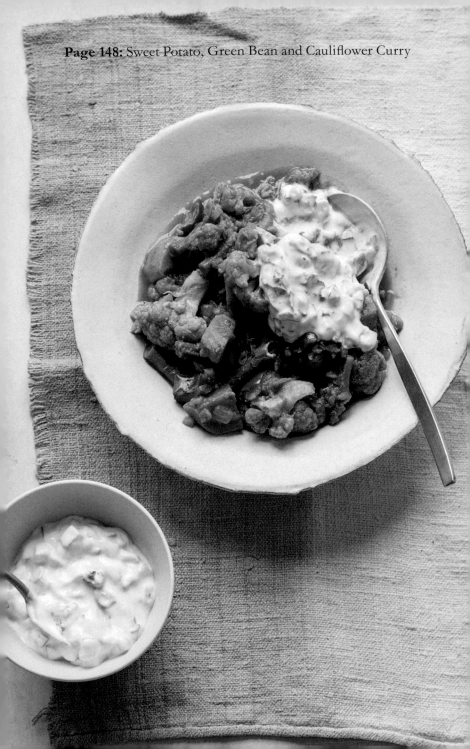

Page 148: Sweet Potato, Green Bean and Cauliflower Curry

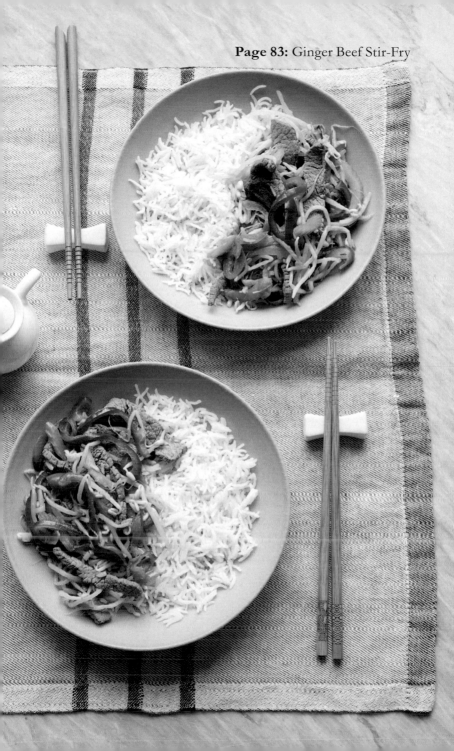

Page 83: Ginger Beef Stir-Fry

Page 152: Rich Mushroom Tagliatelle

then rinse out the food processor or blender with a little of the stock and add to the bowl.

In a non-stick pan sprayed with rapeseed oil, fry the onion until soft. Add the paste and cook for 2 minutes, stirring continuously.

Add the remaining ingredients (except the fresh coriander) and simmer gently for 15 minutes until the sauce thickens and the prawns are cooked through.

Just before serving, stir in the fresh coriander. Serve with the boiled rice.

Arrabbiata Prawns with Rice

Serves 2
Per serving: 292 calories, 0.7g fat
Prep 10 minutes
Cook 25 minutes

This recipe can also be used as a delicious topping for jacket potatoes.

- 110g basmati rice
- 1 vegetable stock cube
- rapeseed oil spray
- ½ red onion, finely chopped
- 1 clove of garlic, crushed
- 1 red pepper, deseeded and finely diced
- 110g raw peeled prawns
- ½ x 400g tin of chopped tomatoes
- ½ fresh red chilli, deseeded and finely chopped
- freshly ground black pepper
- 4–6 fresh basil leaves, to garnish

Cook the rice in boiling water with a vegetable stock cube according to the packet instructions. When cooked, drain well and keep hot.

Heat a non-stick frying pan sprayed with rapeseed oil and fry the onion until soft. Add the garlic and red pepper and cook for a further 2 to 3 minutes. Add the prawns and cook for 5 to 6 minutes.

Add the tomatoes and chilli, bringing the sauce to a gentle simmer. The prawns should be firm and cooked through.

Season with freshly ground black pepper to taste. Add the torn basil leaves and serve with the boiled rice.

Sardine and Tomato Tagliatelle

Serves 2
Per serving: 260 calories, 4.5g fat
Prep 5 minutes
Cook 20 minutes

This sardine and tomato sauce can be frozen.

- 100g tagliatelle
- 1 vegetable stock cube
- 1 baby leek, finely chopped
- 1 clove of garlic, crushed
- rapeseed oil spray
- ½ x 120g tin of sardines in tomato sauce
- ½ x 400g tin of chopped tomatoes
- ½ teaspoon vegetable stock powder
- 1 tablespoon chopped fresh basil, plus extra to garnish
- freshly ground black pepper
- cherry tomatoes, to garnish

Cook the pasta in a pan of boiling water containing the vegetable stock cube, according to the packet instructions.

Place the leek and garlic in a large non-stick pan sprayed with rapeseed oil and cook until soft. Stir in the sardines, chopped tomatoes and stock powder and simmer to allow the tomatoes to reduce, seasoning with black pepper. Add the chopped basil and reduce the heat.

Drain the pasta and transfer to serving bowls. Remove the sauce from the heat, spoon the sauce on top and garnish with cherry tomatoes and the remaining fresh basil.

Tandoori Salmon with Spicy Noodles

Serves 2
Per serving: 383 calories, 6.5% fat (excluding
   accompaniments)
Prep 5 minutes
Cook 10 minutes

- 2 salmon fillets
- 2 teaspoons tandoori curry powder
- 200g straight-to-wok cooked rice noodles
- 2 tablespoons spicy Szechuan sauce
- freshly ground black pepper

Preheat the oven to 200°C/400°F/gas 6.

Roll the salmon fillets in the curry powder and season with the pepper, then place on a non-stick baking tray.

Bake for 6 to 8 minutes until just cooked or microwave for 2 minutes on high heat and allow to stand for 1 minute.

Meanwhile, heat a non-stick pan and stir-fry the rice noodles with the Szechuan sauce until heated through.

Serve the salmon on a bed of noodles with stir-fry vegetables on the side.

VEGETARIAN AND VEGAN

Citrus and Ginger Pappardelle Stir-Fry (vegan)

Serves 2
Per serving: 430 calories, 1.9g fat
Prep 10 minutes
Cook 15 minutes

This is an ideal way of using up packet ends of all types of pastas.

- 130g pappardelle or ribbon pasta
- 1 vegetable stock cube
- 150ml orange juice
- 4 spring onions
- 1 clove of garlic, crushed
- 1 red pepper, deseeded and thinly sliced
- rapeseed oil spray
- 60g mangetout, topped and tailed
- 2.5cm piece of fresh ginger, peeled and finely chopped
- 1 teaspoon light soy sauce
- juice of ½ lime
- freshly ground black pepper

Cook the pasta in a pan of boiling water containing the vegetable stock cube, according to the packet instructions. Drain, return the pasta to the pan and pour the orange juice over.

Meanwhile, place the spring onion, garlic and pepper in a large non-stick pan sprayed with rapeseed oil and cook for 1 to 2 minutes.

Add the mangetout and ginger and continue to cook over a high heat for a further minute.

Pour in the pasta and juice, add the soy and lime juice and toss all the ingredients together. Season with black pepper if required.

Once the pasta is heated through, transfer to a warmed serving dish and serve immediately.

Quorn, Pepper and Mushrooms Stir-Fry (vegan)

Serves 2
Per serving: 400 calories, 0.7% fat
Prep 5 minutes
Cook 30 minutes

- 110g basmati rice
- 1 vegetable stock cube
- 1 red onion, thinly sliced
- 200g Quorn fillets, cut into strips
- rapeseed oil spray
- 2 sticks of celery, sliced
- 1 orange pepper, deseeded and sliced
- 1 red pepper, deseeded and sliced
- 50g button mushrooms
- juice of 1 lime
- 2 tablespoons soy sauce
- 275g bean sprouts

Cook the rice in boiling water with a vegetable stock cube according to the packet instructions. When cooked, drain well and keep hot.

Place the onion and Quorn strips in a large non-stick pan sprayed with rapeseed oil and cook until soft.

Add the celery, peppers and mushrooms along with the lime juice. Toss well, add the soy sauce and cook for 5 minutes.

Just before serving, add the bean sprouts and toss well. Serve with the rice.

Stir-Fried Vegetables with Ginger and Sesame Sauce (vegan)

Serves 2
Per serving: 345 calories, 5.5g fat
Prep 10 minutes
Cook 15 minutes

- 110g basmati rice
- 1 vegetable stock cube
- 1 tablespoon sunflower oil
- 1 onion, sliced
- 175g mangetout, topped and tailed
- 1 small red pepper, deseeded and cut into strips
- 1 small Chinese leaf, shredded
- 200g bean sprouts

for the sauce

- 3 tablespoons fresh ginger juice (see note)
- 1 tablespoon arrowroot
- 3 tablespoons tamari
- 1 teaspoon toasted sesame oil
- 75ml light stock or water

Make the sauce by mixing all the ingredients together thoroughly.

Cook the rice in boiling water with a vegetable stock cube according to the packet instructions. When cooked, drain well and keep hot.

Meanwhile, heat the oil in a wok and quickly fry the onion until soft. Add the mangetout and cook for about 1 minute, stirring continuously to stop them from going brown. Add the red pepper and cook for a further minute.

Add the Chinese leaf and cook until tender, stirring from time to time.

Pour the sauce over the vegetables and bring the mixture back to the boil, then add the bean sprouts. Continue to toss the vegetables for a further 3 to 4 minutes over a low heat.

Serve the rice topped with the vegetable mixture.

Note: To make the ginger juice, use unpeeled fresh root ginger. Grate the ginger and squeeze out as much of the juice as possible.

Broccoli and Pepper Stir-Fry with Noodles (vegan)

Serves 2
Per serving: 298 calories, 5.4g fat (excluding accompaniments)
Prep 10 minutes
Marinate 10 minutes
Cook 15 minutes

- 110g broccoli florets, broken into bite-sized pieces
- 1 red pepper, deseeded and sliced into thin strips
- 110g Chinese noodles
- rapeseed oil spray
- 110g bean sprouts

for the marinade

- ½ red onion, thinly sliced
- 1 clove of garlic, crushed
- 2.5cm piece of fresh ginger, peeled and finely chopped
- 2 tablespoons orange juice
- 1 tablespoon light soy sauce
- 1 teaspoon sesame seeds
- 1 teaspoon finely chopped fresh chilli

Combine all the marinade ingredients in a large bowl. Add the broccoli and pepper to the marinade and mix well. Leave for 10 minutes.

Meanwhile, place the noodles in a heatproof bowl and cover with boiling water. Allow them to stand for 5 minutes.

Heat a large non-stick pan or wok and spray with rapeseed oil. Remove the vegetables from the marinade, reserving the marinade. Stir-fry the marinated vegetables for 5 to 6 minutes until they start to soften. Add the bean sprouts and cook for a further 2 minutes.

Drain the noodles and place in a saucepan. Add the reserved marinade and bring to the boil, combining well.

Serve the vegetables and noodles immediately with a side salad.

Stir-Fried Mushrooms and Peppers (vegan)

Serves 2
Per serving: 46 calories, 0.7g fat
Prep 20 minutes
Cook 10 minutes

A colourful side dish suitable for meat or fish. For added flavour, add 1 or 2 crushed cloves of garlic to the pan during cooking.

- 1 red pepper, deseeded and cut into 2.5cm cubes
- 1 yellow pepper, deseeded and cut into 2.5cm cubes
- 115g button mushrooms
- zest and juice of ½ lemon
- 1 tablespoon light soy sauce
- 1 tablespoon chopped fresh chives

Place the peppers and mushrooms in a bowl.

Pour the lemon zest and juice and the soy sauce over and toss well to coat the vegetables.

Heat a large non-stick wok or pan until hot. Add the vegetables and cook quickly over a high heat, tossing them so that they cook evenly.

Pile into a serving dish and sprinkle with chopped chives.

Chickpea and Root Vegetable Stew with Couscous (vegan)

Serves 2
Per serving: 281 calories, 1.1% fat
Prep 10 minutes
Cook 40 minutes

You can turn this recipe into a chunky soup by adding extra vegetable stock.

- 1 red onion, diced
- 1 clove of garlic, crushed
- rapeseed oil spray
- 2 carrots, peeled and diced
- 100g swede, peeled and diced
- 1 x 400g tin of chickpeas, drained
- 200ml vegetable stock
- 1 small fresh red chilli, thinly sliced
- 1 tablespoon chopped fresh basil
- ½ teaspoon ground cumin
- 1 x 400g tin of chopped tomatoes
- 1 piece of orange zest
- 100g couscous
- freshly ground black pepper
- optional: chopped fresh parsley, to garnish

Place the onion and garlic in a large non-stick pan sprayed with rapeseed oil and cook until soft, then add the vegetables and chickpeas.

Gradually stir in the stock, then add the chilli, basil and cumin.

Stir in the tomatoes and orange zest and allow to simmer gently for 30 minutes, topping up with more water if required, until the vegetables are cooked and the sauce has thickened.

Meanwhile, prepare the couscous according to the packet instructions.

Just before serving, remove the orange zest from the chickpea stew.

Serve hot with couscous and sprinkle with parsley.

Vegetable Chilli (vegan)

Serves 4
Per serving: 402 calories, 1.4g fat
Prep 10 minutes
Cook 1 hour

This is the simplest of recipes, ideal for entertaining and perfect for freezing.

- 1 x 400g tin of tomatoes
- 1 x 210g tin of red kidney beans, rinsed and drained
- 1 teaspoon tomato purée
- 2 teaspoons sweet pickle or Branston Pickle
- 1 clove of garlic, crushed
- 1 eating apple, peeled and chopped
- 1 onion, chopped
- 100g broad beans
- 100g peas
- 1 large carrot, chopped
- 100g sweet potatoes, peeled and chopped
- 1 teaspoon chilli powder
- 3 fresh chillies, deseeded and finely chopped
- 120ml vegetable stock
- 1 bay leaf
- 220g basmati rice
- 1 vegetable stock cube

Place all the ingredients except the rice and stock cube in a saucepan and cover with a lid. Simmer for 50 minutes over a low heat, stirring occasionally.

Cook the rice in boiling water with a vegetable stock

cube according to the packet instructions. When cooked, drain well and keep hot.

After 50 minutes, remove the lid and continue to cook until the liquid is reduced and the mixture is of a thick consistency.

Serve the chilli with the rice.

Spicy Chickpea Casserole (vegan)

Serves 2
Per serving: 320 calories, 7.6g fat
Prep 25 minutes
Cook 40 minutes

- 2 leeks, finely chopped
- 2 courgettes, diced
- 3 sticks of celery, chopped
- rapeseed oil spray
- ½ teaspoon ground cumin
- ½ teaspoon ground turmeric
- ½ teaspoon five spice
- 2 cloves of garlic, chopped
- 2 teaspoons chopped fresh oregano
- 1 x 400g tin of chickpeas, rinsed
- 600ml vegetable stock
- 2 teaspoons cornflour
- freshly ground black pepper
- optional: 2 pieces of orange zest, finely shredded, to garnish
- optional: finely shredded courgette strips, to garnish

Place the leek, courgette and celery in a large non-stick pan sprayed with rapeseed oil and cook for 2 to 3 minutes until lightly coloured.

Add the spices, garlic and oregano and continue to cook for 1 minute. Add the chickpeas to the pan.

Add the stock, bring the mixture to a gentle simmer and cook for 30 minutes.

Stir the cornflour in a small bowl or jug with a little cold water and mix to a smooth paste.

Stir the slaked cornflour into the casserole and simmer gently for another 5 minutes.

Garnish with the orange zest and courgette strips.

Chilli Beans (vegan)

Serves 4
Per serving: 163 calories, 2.7g fat (excluding accompaniments)
Prep 10 minutes
Cook 25 minutes

This is a wholesome, hearty meal, which is full of flavour
and goodness and could not be easier to make. It will
keep for up to 5 days in the fridge and can be used as a
soup for lunch or as a dinner.

- 1 red onion, finely chopped
- 1 small fresh red chilli, sliced
- rapeseed oil spray
- ½ x 400g tin of chickpeas, drained and rinsed
- ½ x 400g tin of red kidney beans, drained and rinsed
- 1 x 400g tin of chopped tomatoes
- 600ml vegetable stock (use 2 vegetable stock cubes)
- 1 tablespoon tomato purée
- 2 teaspoon chopped fresh oregano
- freshly ground black pepper

Place the onion and chilli in a large non-stick pan
sprayed with rapeseed oil and cook for 3 to 4 minutes.

Transfer to a saucepan and add the remaining ingredients. Simmer gently for 20 minutes.

Season to taste with pepper and serve.

Blackeye Beans with Ginger and Soy (vegan)

Serves 2
Per serving: 373 calories, 3.8g fat
Prep 20 minutes
Cook 45 minutes

Fresh ginger and soy sauce add a slightly Asian theme to this dish. As a variation, try serving it with rice mixed with fresh bean sprouts.

- 50g blackeye beans
- 2 vegetable stock cubes
- 100g basmati rice
- ½ onion, diced
- 175g mushrooms, sliced
- 1 stick of celery, cut into thin strips
- 1 carrot, cut into thin strips
- 50g water chestnuts, thinly sliced
- ½ teaspoon chilli powder
- ½ teaspoon grated fresh ginger or ground ginger
- 1 clove of garlic, crushed
- 150ml vegetable stock
- 1 tablespoon soy sauce
- 15g cornflour
- freshly ground black pepper

Place the blackeye beans in plenty of water in a saucepan with a vegetable stock cube. Cover, bring to the boil and simmer for 30 to 35 minutes. Drain well.

Cook the rice in boiling water with a vegetable stock

cube according to the packet instructions. When cooked, drain well and keep hot.

Meanwhile, in a separate pan gently heat the vegetables, chestnuts, chilli, ginger and garlic in a little of the vegetable stock.

Mix the soy sauce and cornflour with a little vegetable stock, add the remainder of the stock and stir into the vegetables, stirring continuously.

Add the drained beans and simmer for a further 8 to 10 minutes. Season to taste with the pepper and serve with the rice.

Aubergine Tagine with Couscous (vegan)

Serves 2
Per serving: 255 calories, 0.5% fat
Prep 10 minutes
Cook 30 minutes

Cook this dish slowly over a low heat for maximum flavour.

- 1 large red onion, finely diced
- 1 clove of garlic, crushed
- rapeseed oil spray
- 1 aubergine, diced
- 2 teaspoons tagine paste
- ½ x 400g tin of chopped tomatoes
- 75ml fresh orange juice
- 1 teaspoon stock powder
- 100g couscous
- freshly ground black pepper
- optional: fresh mint, to garnish

Place the onion and garlic in a large non-stick pan sprayed with rapeseed oil and cook until soft.

Add the aubergine and tagine paste and continue to cook to brown the aubergine.

Add the tomatoes, orange juice, stock powder and pepper. Cover with a lid and simmer gently for 25 minutes, adding more stock if required.

Meanwhile, prepare the couscous according to the packet instructions.

Serve the tagine with the couscous and garnished with mint.

Baked Aubergine with Chickpeas, Bulgur and Feta-Style Cheese (vegan)

Serves 2
Per serving: 403 calories, 2.2% fat
Prep 10 minutes
Cook 1 hour

- 2 medium aubergines
- 60g bulgur wheat
- 1 small red onion
- rapeseed oil spray
- 1 clove of garlic, finely diced
- 1 x 210g tin of chickpeas, drained
- 1 x 210g tin of kidney beans, drained
- ¼ teaspoon ground cinnamon
- ¼ teaspoon chilli powder
- 50g feta-style plant-based cheese
- salt and freshly ground black pepper
- finely chopped fresh mint, to garnish

Preheat the oven to 190°C/375°F/gas 5.

Place a cut along the length of each aubergine, about a quarter of the way through. Lay the aubergines, cut side down, on a lined baking tray and roast in the oven for about 45 minutes until the flesh is tender.

In the meantime, place the bulgur wheat into a bowl and cover with boiling water. Set aside for 25 to 35 minutes until the grains have softened and the liquid absorbed.

Peel the onion, cutting a few slices for garnish, then dice the remainder.

Ten minutes before the aubergines are due to come out

of the oven, heat a non-stick frying pan and spray with rapeseed oil. Put the diced onion and garlic in the pan and cook gently for 5 to 7 minutes until softened.

Add the drained chickpeas and kidney beans, plus the cinnamon and chilli powder to the pan and cook for a further 2 to 3 minutes.

Drain any excess water away from the bulgur wheat and add the grains to the frying pan. Stir gently to heat through and season with a little salt and freshly ground black pepper. Remove from the heat.

Remove the aubergines from the oven. Using two forks, gently push the flesh to the sides to make room for the filling. Carefully divide the chickpea and bulgur filling between the two aubergines. Crumble over the feta-style cheese. Top with the reserved sliced onion and chopped fresh mint. Serve immediately.

Lentil and Roast Vegetable Loaf (vegetarian)

Serves 4
Per serving: 258 calories, 4.8g fat
Prep 25 minutes
Cook 1 hour 10 minutes

A vegan meatloaf that is delicious served with green vegetables or a side salad.

- 2 onions, finely chopped
- 2 courgettes, diced
- 1 small aubergine, diced
- 1 large red pepper, deseeded and diced
- 175g red lentils
- 1 x 400g tin of chopped tomatoes
- 150ml vegetable stock
- 2 cloves of garlic, crushed
- 2 teaspoons chopped fresh thyme
- 2 eggs, beaten
- freshly ground black pepper
- fresh basil, to garnish

Preheat the oven to 200°C/400°F/gas 6.

Place the prepared vegetables into a roasting tin, season well with black pepper and bake at the top of the oven for 25 to 30 minutes until lightly roasted.

Meanwhile, in a saucepan bring to the boil the lentils, tomatoes, stock, garlic and thyme. Simmer for 15 minutes to soften the lentils and allow them to absorb the liquid.

Mix the lentil mixture with the vegetables in a mixing bowl, adding the beaten egg.

Pour the mixture into a lightly greased 1kg (2 lb) loaf tin and stand in a roasting tin containing 2 to 3cm water. Bake in the middle of the oven for 40 minutes until risen and set. Allow to cool slightly before serving.

Just before serving, sprinkle with fresh basil.

Note: Although the loaf can be served straight from the oven, it is best if allowed to cool and set completely, and then reheated as required either as a whole or sliced.

Roast Vegetable and Lentil Dhal (vegan)

Serves 2
Per serving: 220 calories, 1.8g fat
Prep 25 minutes
Cook 40 minutes

- 1 onion, finely chopped
- 1 courgette, diced
- ½ small aubergine, diced
- 1 small red pepper, deseeded and diced
- 90g red lentils
- ½ x 400g tin of chopped tomatoes
- 75ml vegetable stock
- 1 clove of garlic, crushed
- 1 teaspoon chopped fresh thyme
- 1 teaspoon garam masala powder
- 4 cardamom pods, crushed and seeds removed
- freshly ground black pepper
- optional: fresh mint, to garnish

Preheat the oven to 200°C/400°F/gas 6.

Place the prepared vegetables into a roasting tin, season well with black pepper and bake at the top of the oven for 25 to 30 minutes until lightly roasted.

Meanwhile, in a large saucepan bring to the boil the lentils, tomatoes, stock, garlic, thyme and spices.

Simmer for 15 to 20 minutes to soften the lentils and allow them to absorb the liquid.

Add the roasted vegetables and simmer for 10 minutes more to allow the flavours to combine.

Just before serving, sprinkle with fresh mint.

Roasted Vegetable Curry (vegan)

Serves 2
Per serving: 353 calories, 5.6g fat
Prep 15 minutes
Cook 45 minutes

This curry is so easy to make because you simply roast the vegetables first, then add to the sauce. Try with any combination of vegetables. For a creamy curry, stir in 2 tablespoons of virtually fat-free fromage frais (or plant-based alternative) just before serving.

- ½ small aubergine, diced
- 1 red pepper, deseeded and diced
- 1 yellow pepper, deseeded and diced
- ½ red onion, chopped
- 1 courgette, sliced
- 6 cherry tomatoes
- 1 clove of garlic, crushed
- ½ tablespoon mild curry powder
- 1 tablespoon light soy sauce
- 300g tomato passata
- 4 cardamom pods, crushed and seeds removed
- 110g basmati rice
- 1 vegetable stock cube
- freshly ground black pepper
- 1 tablespoon chopped fresh coriander, to garnish

Preheat the oven to 200°C/400°F/gas 6.
Place all the vegetables in a roasting tin and season well

with freshly ground black pepper. Dot with crushed garlic and sprinkle the curry powder over.

Drizzle with the soy sauce and place in the top of the oven. Roast for 20 to 25 minutes until the vegetables start to soften.

In a large saucepan, heat the passata with the cardamom and add the cooked vegetables. Simmer over a low heat for 15 minutes to allow the sauce to thicken.

Cook the rice in boiling water with a vegetable stock cube according to the packet instructions. When cooked, drain well and keep hot.

Check the seasoning of the curry, add the fresh coriander and serve with the rice.

Sweet Potato, Green Bean and Cauliflower Curry (vegan)

Serves 2
Per serving: 436 calories, 2.6g fat (excluding accompaniments)
Prep 15 minutes
Cook 30 minutes

- 110g basmati rice
- 1 vegetable stock cube
- 1 small onion, chopped
- 1 clove of garlic, crushed
- 1 fresh green chilli, finely chopped
- 2.5cm piece of fresh ginger, finely chopped
- rapeseed oil spray
- 150ml vegetable stock
- 1 teaspoon garam masala
- ½ teaspoon ground coriander
- ½ teaspoon ground cumin
- 225g sweet potatoes, cut into 2.5cm chunks
- 120g green beans, trimmed and cut into 2.5cm lengths
- 225g cauliflower, broken into small florets
- ½ red pepper, deseeded and cut into small pieces
- 150g tomato passata
- 1 banana

Cook the rice in boiling water with a vegetable stock cube according to the packet instructions. When cooked, drain well and keep hot.

Place the onion, garlic, chilli and ginger in a large non-stick pan sprayed with rapeseed oil, cover with a lid and fry for 5 minutes over a gentle heat. Add a little of the vegetable stock if the pan becomes too dry.

When the onion is soft, add 50ml of the stock, sprinkle the spices into the pan and cook for a further minute, stirring continuously. Add the sweet potato, beans, cauliflower and red pepper to the pan and cook over a moderate heat for 2 to 3 minutes, stirring continuously. Pour in the remaining vegetable stock and the passata. Cover the pan and cook gently for 10 minutes.

Slice the banana and add to the pan. Cook for a further 10 minutes or until the vegetables are tender.

Serve with the rice and raita made from low-fat natural yoghurt mixed with chopped cucumber and a little fresh mint.

Quorn Thai Red Curry (vegan)

Serves 2
Per serving: 308 calories, 2.4g fat
Prep 10 minutes
Cook 20 minutes

- 110g basmati rice
- 1 vegetable stock cube
- 1 red onion, finely chopped
- 1 clove of garlic, crushed
- rapeseed oil spray
- 150g fresh or frozen Quorn pieces
- ½ teaspoon ground coriander
- 1 teaspoon finely chopped lemongrass
- 1 red pepper, deseeded and thinly sliced
- 300g tomato passata
- 1 small fresh red chilli, thinly sliced
- optional: 1 kaffir lime leaf
- freshly ground black pepper
- 1 tablespoon chopped fresh coriander, to garnish

Cook the rice in boiling water with a vegetable stock cube according to the packet instructions. When cooked, drain well and keep hot.

Place the onion and garlic in a large non-stick pan sprayed with rapeseed oil and cook until soft. Add the Quorn pieces and season well with black pepper. Stir in the ground coriander and lemongrass.

Add the red pepper, passata, chilli and lime leaf, if using, and bring to a simmer. Reduce the heat and allow

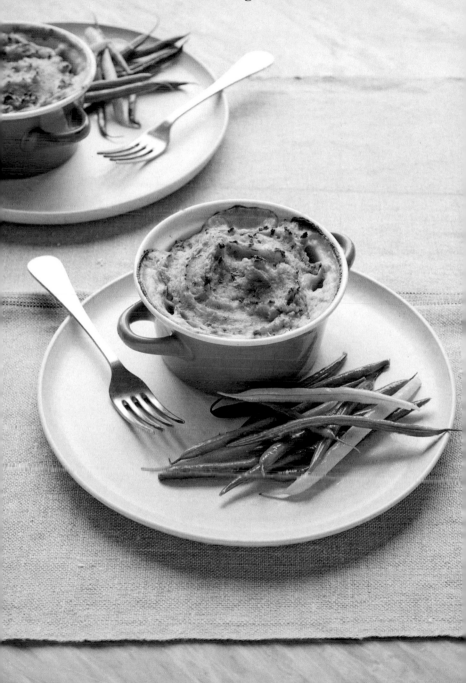

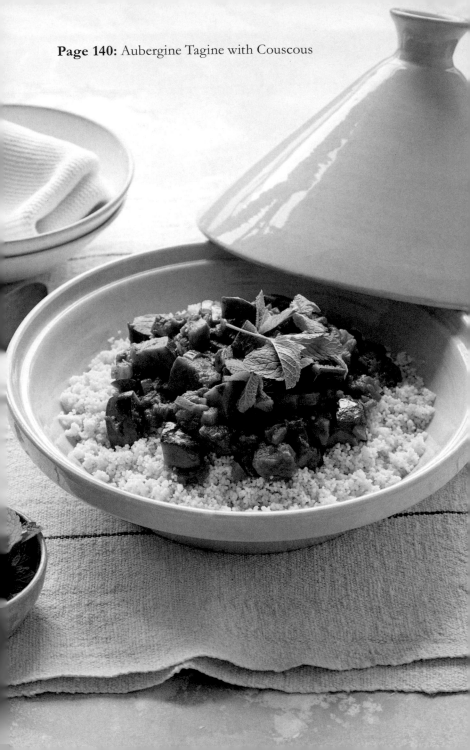

Page 140: Aubergine Tagine with Couscous

Page 163: Stuffed Mushrooms

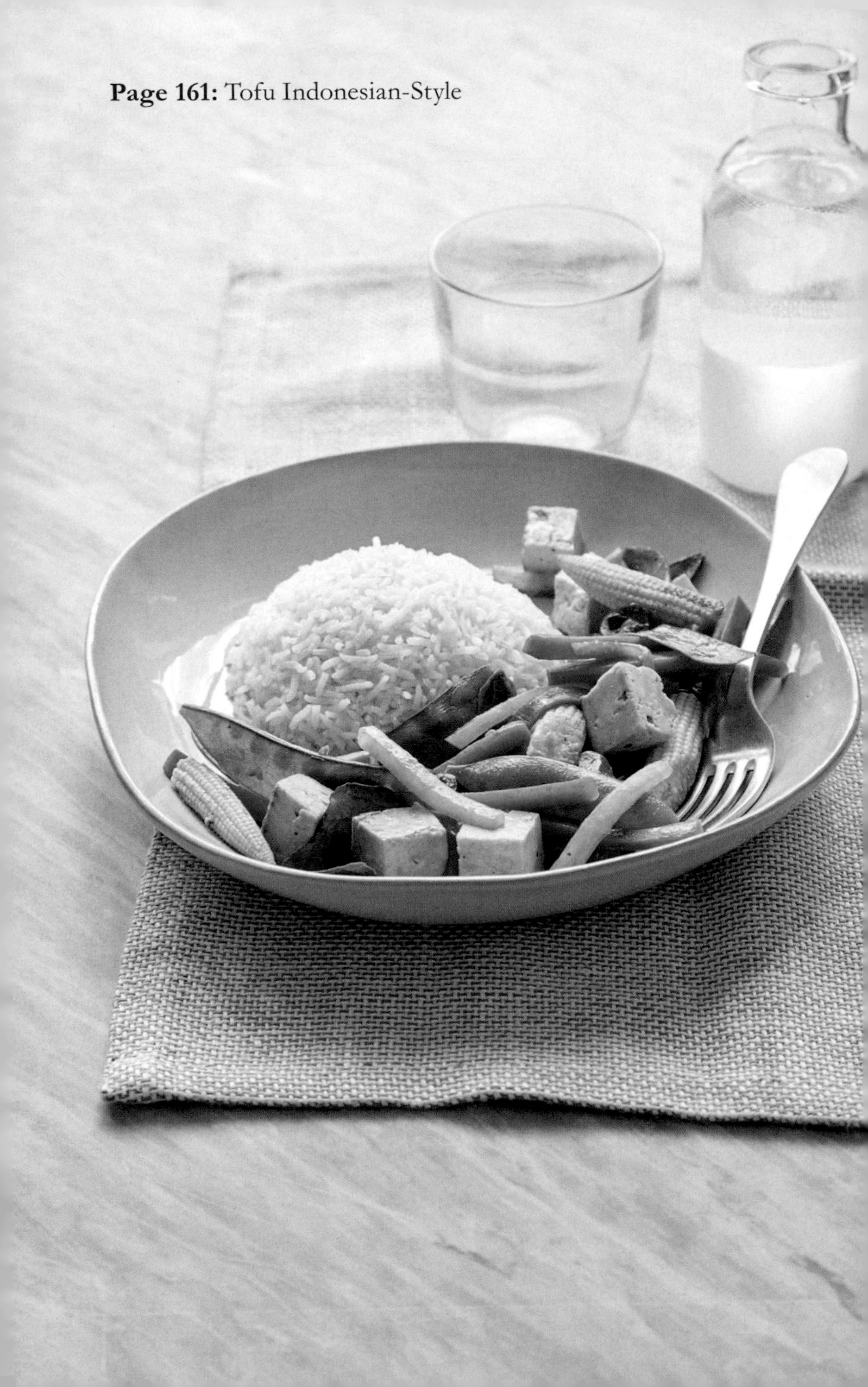

Page 161: Tofu Indonesian-Style

Page 141: Baked Aubergine with Chickpeas, Bulgur and Feta-Style Cheese

Page 110: Spicy Lemon Chicken

Page 87: Beef and Ale Stew

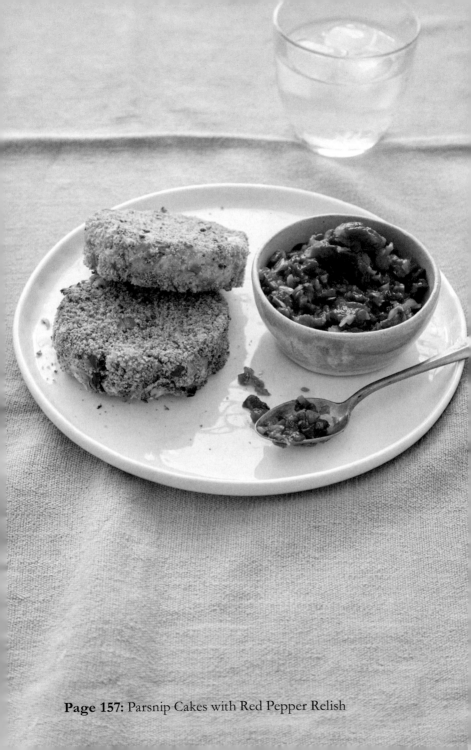

Page 157: Parsnip Cakes with Red Pepper Relish

to simmer for 10 minutes until the sauce has reduced slightly.

Add the chopped fresh coriander to the curry and serve with the rice.

Rich Mushroom Tagliatelle (vegetarian)

Serves 1
Per serving: 390 calories, 1% fat
Prep 5 minutes
Cook 25 minutes

- 70g tagliatelle
- 1 small clove of garlic, finely diced
- ¼ teaspoon chia seeds
- 180g mixed mushrooms
- rapeseed oil spray
- 125ml medium white wine
- 1 tablespoon mushroom ketchup
- 1 teaspoon white miso paste
- optional: fresh herbs, such as chopped chives, to garnish

Cook the pasta in a pan of boiling water according to the packet instructions.

Place the garlic, chia seeds and mushrooms in a large non-stick pan sprayed with rapeseed oil and cook until the mushrooms start to soften.

Add the white wine, mushroom ketchup and the miso paste to the frying pan and stir to combine, then reduce the heat to a gentle simmer. If the liquid reduces so that it's dry, add a little of the pasta water – 1 tablespoon at a time – so that you have a light sauce.

Once the pasta is cooked, remove from the heat and drain carefully.

Transfer the pasta to a warmed plate or bowl and top with the mushroom mixture. Garnish with a few fresh herbs such as chopped chives and serve immediately.

Roast Vegetable and Chickpea Pasta (vegan)

Serves 2
Per serving: 342 calories, 5g fat
Prep 5 minutes
Cook 30 minutes

- ½ red onion, diced
- 1 clove of garlic, chopped
- 1 small courgette, diced
- 1 leek, diced
- 1 red pepper, deseeded and diced
- ½ x 400g tin of chickpeas, drained
- 1 tablespoon soy sauce
- 90g pasta
- 1 vegetable stock cube
- ½ x 400g tin of chopped tomatoes
- 1 teaspoon low-fat pesto
- freshly ground black pepper

Preheat the oven to 200°C/400°F/gas 6.

Place the onion, garlic, courgette, leek, red pepper and chickpeas into an ovenproof dish. Pour over the soy sauce and season with freshly ground black pepper.

Bake in the oven for 20 minutes until slightly charred.

Meanwhile, cook the pasta in a pan of boiling water containing the vegetable stock cube, according to the packet instructions. Drain and keep warm.

Remove the vegetable mixture from the oven and spoon into a saucepan along with the chopped tomatoes. Mix well. Bring to a gentle simmer and add the pesto.

Serve the pasta with the sauce on top.

Tomato, Basil and Lemon Penne (vegan)

Serves 2
Per serving: 266 calories, 3.9g fat
Prep 10 minutes
Cook 20 minutes

- 225g penne
- 1 vegetable stock cube
- ½ red onion, finely chopped
- rapeseed oil spray
- 1 clove of garlic, crushed
- 1 red pepper, deseeded and thinly sliced
- ½ x 400g tin of chopped tomatoes
- ½ fresh red chilli, deseeded and thinly sliced (or a few dried chilli flakes)
- grated zest of ½ a lemon
- 6–8 fresh basil leaves, shredded
- freshly ground black pepper
- ½ lemon, cut into segments, to serve

Cook the pasta in a pan of boiling water containing the vegetable stock cube, according to the packet instructions.

Place the onion in a large non-stick pan sprayed with rapeseed oil and cook until soft. Add the garlic and red pepper and cook for a further 2 to 3 minutes.

Add the tomatoes, chilli and lemon zest, bring the sauce to a gentle simmer and continue to cook for a further 10 minutes. Season with the pepper.

Drain the pasta and pour into a serving dish. Spoon the sauce over and sprinkle with the basil leaves. Serve with segments of fresh lemon.

Note: The sauce can be frozen.

Marjoram-Stuffed Peppers (vegan)

Serves 2
Per serving: 201 calories, 5.6g fat (excluding accompaniments)
Prep 10 minutes
Cook 45 minutes

These peppers can be made in advance and reheated as required. Red and yellow peppers tend to taste sweeter than green, but if you like the flavour, use all three.

- 60g fresh brown breadcrumbs
- ½ tablespoon chopped fresh marjoram
- 2 red peppers
- 2 yellow peppers
- 2 shallots, finely chopped
- 1 clove of garlic, crushed
- rapeseed oil spray
- 1 x 200g tin of artichoke hearts, drained and chopped
- freshly ground black pepper

Preheat the oven to 200°C/400°F/gas 6.

Scatter the breadcrumbs over the base of a non-stick baking tray. Add the marjoram and season well with black pepper. Bake in the oven for 15 to 20 minutes, turning every so often to prevent the edges from burning.

Meanwhile, slice the tops off the peppers and scoop out and discard the inner seeds. Remove the stalk from the tops and chop the tops very finely.

Place the shallots and garlic in a large non-stick pan sprayed with rapeseed oil and cook until soft. Add the chopped pepper tops and continue to cook for 4 to 5 minutes.

Add the artichoke hearts and toasted breadcrumbs. Mix together all the ingredients and season to taste.

Spoon the filling into the pepper shells and place them side by side in an ovenproof dish. Cover with foil and bake in the centre of the oven for 20 minutes.

Remove the foil and return to the oven for a further 5 minutes to brown.

Serve with new potatoes, in their skins, and either a mixed salad or vegetables.

Parsnip Cakes with Red Pepper Relish
(with vegan option)

Serves 4
Per serving: 290 calories, 3.8g fat (excluding accompaniments)
Prep 20 minutes
Cook 40 minutes

These tasty parsnip cakes can be made in advance and frozen. The relish adds moisture to the finished dish, but as it takes a little time to prepare, you may like to make it in advance.

- 1kg young parsnips, peeled and cut into small pieces
- 1 vegetable stock cube
- 4 small leeks, sliced
- 1 red pepper, deseeded and diced
- rapeseed oil spray
- 1 clove of garlic, crushed
- 2 teaspoons chopped fresh thyme
- 2 tablespoons fromage frais (or plant-based alternative)
- 1 tablespoon finely chopped fresh chives
- 50g fresh brown breadcrumbs
- freshly ground black pepper

for the red pepper relish

- 6 red peppers, halved and deseeded
- 1 red onion, finely chopped
- 1 clove of garlic, crushed
- 2–3 teaspoons chilli sauce

Preheat the oven to 200°C/400°F/gas 6.

Cook the parsnips in a pan of boiling water containing the vegetable stock cube until tender. Drain well and return to the pan. Mash with a potato masher until smooth, adding plenty of black pepper.

Meanwhile, place the leek and red pepper in a large non-stick pan sprayed with rapeseed oil and cook until soft. Add the garlic and thyme, mixing well.

Combine the parsnip and leek mixtures, then add the fromage frais and chives.

When cool, form the mixture into eight potato cake shapes and roll in the fresh breadcrumbs.

Place the cakes on a baking tray and bake near the top of the oven for 10 to 15 minutes until golden brown.

To make the red pepper relish, place the peppers on a non-stick baking tray and roast in the oven for 30 minutes until they are well charred, turning halfway through.

Remove the peppers from the oven and place immediately into a plastic food bag. Seal the bag and allow to cool. When cool, remove the peppers and peel away the skins. Chop the flesh into small dice.

Place the onion and garlic in a large non-stick pan sprayed with rapeseed oil and cook for 2 minutes, then stir in the peppers and chilli sauce. Spoon into a serving bowl.

Serve the parsnip cakes with the relish and accompany with salad or vegetables.

Chilli Pinto Bean Burritos (vegan)

Serves 2
Per serving: 400 calories, 5g fat
Prep 15 minutes
Cook 40 minutes

Pinto beans are beige in colour with brown speckles. They are native to Mexico, but now are mostly grown in the United States.

- 1 red onion, finely chopped
- 1 clove of garlic, crushed
- rapeseed oil spray
- 2 fresh green chillies, deseeded and chopped
- 1 medium courgette, grated
- ½ x 400g tin of pinto beans, drained and rinsed
- ½ x 400g tin of chopped tomatoes
- 150g tomato passata
- 1 teaspoon chopped fresh oregano
- 1½ teaspoons vegetable stock powder
- 2 tortilla wraps
- shredded lettuce, to serve
- chopped spring onion, to serve

Place the onion and garlic in a large non-stick pan sprayed with rapeseed oil and cook for 1 to 2 minutes until soft. Add the chilli and courgette and continue to cook for 2 minutes.

Stir in the beans, tomatoes, passata, oregano and stock powder and bring to the boil. Reduce the heat and cover. Simmer gently for 20 to 25 minutes until the sauce thickens.

Serve as a filling in a tortilla wrap with shredded lettuce and chopped spring onion.

Teriyaki Tempeh with Rice and Broccoli (vegan)

Serves 1
Per serving: 423 calories, 3% fat
Prep 5 minutes
Cook 25 minutes

- 50g basmati rice
- 1 vegetable stock cube
- 70g tempeh, cut into small chunks
- 90g broccoli florets
- rapeseed oil spray
- 1½ tablespoons teriyaki sauce
- ¼ teaspoon flaxseeds
- ¼ teaspoon sesame seeds, to garnish

Cook the rice in boiling water with a vegetable stock cube according to the packet instructions. When cooked, drain well and keep hot.

Steam the tempeh for 6 to 8 minutes with the broccoli florets. Remove the tempeh and broccoli from the steamer, transfer the broccoli to a bowl and keep warm.

Heat a small frying pan and spray with rapeseed oil. Add the steamed tempeh chunks and gently stir-fry for 5 minutes.

Add the teriyaki sauce and flaxseeds to the tempeh with 1 tablespoon of water. Reduce the heat and cook for a further 2 to 3 minutes, stirring gently, then add the broccoli and cook for a further 2 minutes.

Top the rice with the teriyaki tempeh and broccoli. Garnish with the sesame seeds and serve immediately.

Tofu Indonesian-Style (vegan)

Serves 2
Per serving: 350 calories, 6.4g fat
Prep 10 minutes
Cook 20 minutes

- 110g basmati rice
- 1 vegetable stock cube
- 140g regular tofu
- ½ tablespoon sunflower oil
- 100g baby carrots, thinly sliced
- 90g baby sweetcorn, cut in half diagonally
- 90g mangetout, topped and tailed
- 50g turnip or white radish, peeled and thinly sliced
- freshly ground black pepper

for the sauce

- 1 teaspoon arrowroot
- 1 tablespoon tamari (see note)
- 1 kaffir lime leaf or bay leaf
- 1 small fresh chilli, deseeded and sliced
- 1 x 5cm piece of lemongrass
- 1 teaspoon fresh ginger juice (see note)
- 75ml vegetable stock

Cook the rice in boiling water with a vegetable stock cube according to the packet instructions. When cooked, drain well and keep hot.

Cut the tofu into 20 pieces and leave to drain on paper towels.

Heat the oil and sweat the vegetables in a semi-covered pan for 5 minutes, stirring continuously.

Mix all the sauce ingredients together, adding only sufficient vegetable stock to form a smooth sauce. Add the tofu and pour the sauce and tofu over the vegetables. Cover and cook for 8 minutes.

Season to taste, remove the lime or bay leaf and the lemongrass and serve with the rice.

Note: Tamari is a good-quality soy sauce from Japan and is available in many health food shops and in some supermarkets. If you can't find it, you can substitute any soy sauce.

To make the ginger juice, use unpeeled fresh root ginger. Grate the ginger and squeeze out as much of the juice as possible.

Stuffed Mushrooms (vegetarian)

Serves 2
Per serving: 185 calories, 8g fat
Prep 5 minutes
Cook 10 minutes

This is a surprisingly filling lunch.

- 4 very large flat mushrooms, wiped clean
- 1 red onion, finely chopped
- 1 slice of wholegrain bread, made into breadcrumbs
- rapeseed oil spray
- 40g hard cheese, grated
- freshly ground black pepper

Preheat the grill to maximum heat, but lower the shelf slightly.

Remove the stalks from the mushrooms. Chop the stalks finely and place in a bowl. Add the onion and the breadcrumbs and mix well. Season with freshly ground black pepper.

Place the mushrooms on their backs in a grill pan or ovenproof dish and fill with the breadcrumb mixture. Spray with rapeseed oil and top with the grated cheese.

Place the mushrooms under the grill but not too close to the elements to avoid burning. Grill for about 7 to 9 minutes to cook through.

SIDES AND SALADS

Dry-Roasted Sweet Potatoes (vegan)

Serves 1
Per serving: 85 calories, 1g fat
Prep 5 minutes
Cook 50 minutes

Sweet potatoes are more nutritious than normal floury potatoes and taste delicious dry-roasted.

- 1 medium sweet potato per person
- 1 vegetable stock cube

Preheat the oven to 180°C/350°F/gas 4.

Peel the sweet potato and chop in half, or into quarters if larger.

Place the potato in a pan of water with the vegetable stock cube and bring to the boil. Cook for 7 minutes, then remove with a slotted spoon and place on a non-stick baking tray.

Cook at the top of the oven for 35–45 minutes or until tender.

Note: You can dry-roast parsnips in exactly the same way. Just top and tail and peel each parsnip, cutting off the narrow end to 3cm and leave that piece whole. Chop the top half into halves or quarters depending on the size.

Home-Made Coleslaw (vegetarian)

Serves 2
Per serving: 70 calories, 2.1g fat
Prep 10 minutes

- 1 large carrot, peeled and coarsely grated
- 1 red onion, thinly sliced
- ¼ white cabbage, finely shredded
- low-fat mayonnaise or salad cream
- optional: a squeeze of lemon juice
- freshly ground black pepper

Put the carrot, onion and cabbage in a bowl, mix well with the low-fat mayonnaise or salad cream and season with pepper.

Note: This will last for 3 days in a fridge if kept in an airtight container.

Marinated Roast Vegetables (vegan)

Serves 2
Per serving: 130 calories, 3.9g fat
Prep 10 minutes
Marinate 30 minutes
Cook 40 minutes

These marinated roast vegetables are perfect served piping hot from the oven or chilled with salad leaves. Either way, the strong, contrasting flavours make this a very healthy and tasty dish.

- 1 courgette
- 1 small aubergine
- ½ red and ½ yellow pepper, deseeded
- 1 baby leek
- ½ small bulb of fennel
- 1 small red onion
- rapeseed oil spray
- 1 tablespoon sesame seeds
- freshly ground black pepper
- fresh parsley, to garnish

for the marinade

- 2 tablespoons lemon juice
- 1 tablespoon light soy sauce
- 1 teaspoon finely chopped lemongrass
- 1 tablespoon chopped fresh marjoram

Preheat the oven to 180°C/350°F/gas 4.

Prepare the vegetables by slicing into wedges 5mm thick.

Combine all the marinade ingredients in a small bowl.

Place the vegetables into a roasting tin, season well with black pepper and spoon the marinade over the vegetables. Set aside.

After 15 minutes, turn the vegetables to ensure even flavouring. Leave for another 15 minutes, turn again, spray with rapeseed oil and sprinkle with the sesame seeds.

Place in the oven and roast for 35 to 40 minutes until tender and slightly charred around the edges.

Sprinkle with parsley and serve hot or allow to cool and serve cold as a salad.

Salmon Pasta Salad

Serves 2
Per serving: 420 calories, 12.9g fat
Prep 10 minutes
Cook 25 minutes

A cold pasta salad with flakes of pink salmon. If fresh salmon is unavailable, tinned salmon is a good substitute.

- 2 vegetable stock cubes
- 175g fresh salmon fillet
- 110g pasta shapes
- 150ml live natural yoghurt
- juice of ½ lemon
- 1 small red onion, finely chopped
- 1 tablespoon chopped fresh chives
- a pinch of sweet paprika
- chopped fresh dill, to garnish

Finely chop one of the vegetable stock cubes into a large saucepan, add about 200ml water and bring to just boiling.

Add the salmon and poach for 8 to 10 minutes over a low heat. Lift the salmon from the pan and allow to cool.

Meanwhile, cook the pasta in a large saucepan of boiling water with the remaining vegetable stock cube according to the instructions on the packet. When cooked, drain the pasta thoroughly and transfer to a mixing bowl.

When the pasta is cold, stir in the yoghurt, lemon juice, onion, chives and paprika.

Carefully flake the salmon into the bowl, removing any

bones and skin, and gently combine all the ingredients with a large spoon, taking care not to over-mix and break up the salmon too much.

Spoon into a serving dish and chill until required. Garnish with fresh dill.

6. Exercise – Immunity's Best Friend

If you wanted to make a list of the most important factors that help you to stay healthy, then keeping active has to be close to the top. The result of a sedentary lifestyle has a huge effect on the body at any age but much more so as we get older. This 28-Day Immunity Plan is appropriate for all age groups, but even more for those in the older age category as the immune system naturally 'tires' as we age. If ever there was a calling for us to stay as active as we can for as long as we possibly can, then that time is right now. Physical movement not only improves our immunity as we age but also our stamina, muscle strength, flexibility, balance and it even helps us have stronger bones. And yes, this programme has it all!

It's Never Too Late to Start!

If you think you have left it too late, then think again. Starting at the right level for you, and being consistent in your approach by doing it regularly, will reap huge benefits at any age. That is why this programme has a gentle start, allowing the body to gradually get used to the movements and adapt to the exercises in a way that feels safe but at the same time is effective. You will gradually increase your fitness over a period of 28 days with the end result, hopefully, amazing you at your progress. We are encouraging you to invest some time on a daily basis into building and maintaining a stronger body and a more resilient immune system.

Mary and I both teach many people over 65, with most of them in their 70s and some in their 80s. Mary has studied and specialised in this sector. She says: 'I see first-hand the enormous improvement in all aspects of my members' physical and mental health and I am excited that I now have the opportunity to transform the health and fitness of many more through this 28-day immunity booster plan at this challenging time. I have designed this programme to steadily build up your stamina, strength and suppleness in a way which is safe, effective and appropriate to your age, safely and effectively and at the same time strengthen your immune system. It will really work.'

Mary now explains the basis of how she designed this fitness programme and her experiences from running her Trial. Unlike my Trial, when I didn't meet with my trialists because I knew them already, Mary put out an invitation to the general public in her area asking for volunteers. For this and the following two chapters, I am handing over to Mary.

Government activity guidelines for older adults

Adults aged 65 and over should:

- Aim to be physically active every day. Any activity is better than none. The more you do, the better, even if it is just light activity.

- Do activities that improve strength, balance and flexibility on at least 2 days per week.
- Do at least 150 minutes (30 minutes on 5 days) of moderate intensity activity a week or 75 minutes of vigorous intensity activity if you are already active, or a combination of both.
- Reduce time spent sitting or lying down and break up long periods of not moving with some activity.

What counts as moderate activity?

- Brisk walking
- Riding a bike
- Water aerobics and gentle swimming
- Dancing
- Strength training with light hand weights or resistance band
- Pushing a lawnmower
- Hiking

This programme clearly follows all these guidelines and, in fact, for the 28-day period of the Plan it exceeds them, so you get a head start!

What Are the Benefits of This Programme?

Fighting off infection and disease becomes foremost in our minds the older we become. But it doesn't happen on its own. We need to invest effort if we are going to build and maintain a strong immune system. So how do we do that?

A secret army!

Most of us understand that our heart provides a very efficient circulatory system, which pumps blood around our body. We are less aware of our lymphatic system. This is a clever process where our lymphatic system provides a vital role for our immune system. It works by draining excess fluid from bodily tissues and carrying immunity-boosting white blood cells around the body to fight infection. But there is a problem. The lymphatic system does not have a pump and this is where exercise plays such an important role. The movement of our muscles through exercise automatically creates a pump to spread those white blood cells that are so vital in protecting us from infection – like a secret army that's fighting for us. This fact alone should highly motivate us to exercise regularly at any age, but particularly as we get older. This exercise programme is designed to stimulate that system and engage your 'army' to boost your body's ability to fight infection and disease.

Stronger muscles and bones

Muscle is our immune system's best friend! Muscles are unquestionably a key factor in maintaining a stronger immune system as they provide the transport mechanism for our white blood cells to reach where they are needed to fulfil their infection-fighting role. Making them move more and challenging them through exercise will ensure they also help us maintain our ability to carry out our daily tasks and reduce the risk of falls and injury. There really is no downside to exercising and being active.

Sadly, both muscles and bones will degenerate to a significant degree as we age unless we take affirmative action. In someone who does not exercise, the reduction in muscle strength can drop by as much as 40 per cent by the age of 70. In addition, lack of exercise can lead to bones becoming more brittle and less dense, so they are more liable to fracture. Let's arrest that decline right now and start doing exercises that will give you the most benefit.

- **Strengthen your muscles.** For the muscles we are putting special emphasis on the legs so that you can stand up from a chair without assistance, be able to walk upstairs and enjoy going for a walk comfortably and safely. These are vital activities. Also, we will work on building strength in the upper body so you can continue with everyday tasks that help to maintain your independence into your long-term future. There is training for the 'carrying' muscles of the arms and shoulders, the 'pushing' muscles of the chest and the back of the upper arms so you can get out of the bath and get up from the floor in case you fall. All of these activities are important for our everyday lifestyle, but particularly vital if you have grandchildren and you need to get on and off the floor with them!
- **Bones respond well to gentle impact.** By 'impact' we mean a little jump when you land on

your feet with more force, for instance like a gentle pretend-skip. Some of the exercises in this programme include controlled impact exercises that encourage you to land with some force and this effectively strengthens your leg and hip bones. This is not necessarily jumping, which not everyone can manage, but there is encouragement to land heavily to help maintain, or even improve, your bone density.

Boosting stamina

Aerobic exercise is activity that helps you to breathe more deeply and stimulates your heart and lungs. It also burns fat and boosts overall fitness and, importantly, it has a significant and positive effect on our immune system. Just walking on a regular basis has been shown to improve health in the long term. There is a walking element to the programme that encourages you to exercise every day. Significant scientific research recommends that we build up to 150 minutes of aerobic activity a week – that's just 30 minutes a day on 5 days each week. This recommendation is seen as being the optimum amount to maintain health in older age.

Improving posture and balance

As we get older sadly our posture can deteriorate. Unfortunately, postural changes can also present physical problems, which you may have never considered. In extreme cases, breathing is affected and the risk of falling is increased. This workout is designed to strengthen those muscles that have become weak because of an altered posture, and to stretch those muscles that have shortened. For example, round shoulders and a forward head position shorten and tighten the muscles of the chest, whilst the upper back muscles become weak and stretched. The solution is to *lengthen* the chest muscles through stretching and to *strengthen* the upper back muscles with resistance training. This programme also includes the medical 'balance test' of being able to stand on one leg, which is very challenging at first, but it is a trainable activity that significantly improves with practice. The aim is to balance for 30 seconds on each leg. All of these exercises are covered in this programme.

Tips for moving more every day

- Avoid sitting for long periods of time. Every hour, get up and move.
- Try to walk the short car journeys. Many car journeys are under one mile.
- Park further away. Car journeys are often unavoidable but plan more walking around a car journey.
- Walk and talk. Arrange a chat with a friend to include a walk in the park.
- Get outdoors at every opportunity. Breathing outdoor air stimulates the immune system.
- Play music when exercising. You will be more motivated.
- View housework as an exercise routine.

Starting the Exercise Trial

This Trial differs significantly from Rosemary's group. Firstly, Rosemary's group were all known to her over a number of years from her diet and fitness classes, where weight management is a very key element. Her trialists volunteered to be included in the group to give them motivation to lose the weight they had gained during lockdown plus, hopefully, more. Secondly, because they were attending Rosemary's weekly exercise sessions before the pandemic hit, they were already used to regular exercise. However, Rosemary knew that giving them a formal programme to follow on a daily basis would be a useful tool in keeping them fit, and she knew they would be burning some extra calories to help them lose weight more easily.

My group were totally different. My trialists were unknown to me and I particularly selected them as they were not currently following any formal exercise programme and were relatively unfit. I wanted to test how much their overall fitness could improve in just 28 days. I also recognised that by getting them moving and exercising, they would be making a significant difference to their immune system.

Recruiting the trialists

When I was deciding to run this Trial, I knew I had to meet the trialists in person to be able to test them and then measure their progress. Lockdown was only just easing so I decided that I would set up my 'testing station' in my garden and organise for them to visit within very strict time slots. It was certainly a logistical challenge!

The aim was to put the exercise programme to the test over 28 days. The trialists would have to undergo a full fitness test before the start of the Plan and then be tested again at the end.

In the hope of finding suitable volunteers, I put out a request in our local community media for anyone in the 60+ age group who wanted to improve their body's immunity, their fitness and lose a few pounds to contact me. Within a couple of days over 70 people had applied! I was amazed at the response. I thought it was interesting that so many people were very keen to improve their health and fitness and acknowledge that they needed to do more than they were currently doing.

I decided that 12 trialists would be the optimum that would be manageable so, in the end, I enlisted 9 women and 3 men, including two husband and wife teams. I was keen to have some couples within the group as I hoped they would encourage each other, and so Marjory, Jan, Chris, Ann, Jen, Mark, Alva and Anne, plus couples Peter and Jenny and Roger and Lyn, popped round for their 'start' fitness test.

The Fitness Test – What Was Tested?

Lower Body Strength using the 'sit to stand'

This is the standard test to challenge the strength of the legs with both the quadriceps (front thigh muscles) and the gluteal muscles (back of hip) being challenged by standing up and sitting down again for 30 seconds. It is important to realise that our lower body strength is the king of independent living.

Upper Body Strength with arm curls using hand weights

Holding a 2.5kg (5lb) hand weight (ladies) or a 4kg (8lb) weight (men) in one arm, sit on a chair and lower the arm so that it's straight, then lift to the shoulder and lower again. This test is to see how many you can do in 30 seconds. Most people are unaware of the need to exercise the upper body and underestimate its importance in our general everyday living.

Stamina with a 2-minute step test

Stepping on the spot for just 2 minutes sounds very easy until you put it to the test yourself. The knees have to come fairly high and you are encouraged to step as quickly as possible. After the first minute you begin to recognise that you need to breathe more deeply in order to keep up the pace. It is a proper stamina challenge!

Lower Body Flexibility with a 'sit and reach' test

Sitting on the edge of a chair with one leg out straight, leaning forward with both hands, reaching forward to try and reach the toes, keeping the leg straight. The aim is to see how far you are away from the toes or how far you go beyond the toes. This is only tested on one leg and tests flexibility in our hips.

Upper Body Flexibility using the 'back scratch' test

This entails taking one hand behind the shoulder and as far down your back as you can then taking the other arm under and behind to try and get the two hands to connect to touch your middle fingers. The distance is measured either how far away the fingers are from each other or how far past the fingers you can reach. Only one side is tested, and in most people, there is a big difference between each side. This tests the flexibility in our shoulders.

Balance with the ability to stand on one leg for 30 seconds

This is a hard test, but the good news is that you can train your balance and in time you should be able to reach 30 seconds without needing to reach for support.

Body Composition using a Tanita Body Composition Analyzer

This is a special set of scales that does much more than just weigh you. It gives you your Body Mass Index (BMI), which is calculated on your height-to-weight ratio, letting you know where you fall in the range of 'healthy', 'over-weight' or 'obese'. If your BMI is between 20–24.9 you are in the 'healthy' range, 25–29.9 indicates that you are in the 'overweight' range, but if you go above 30, you are defined as being 'obese'. It also does much more than that. It tells you your 'muscle-to-fat' ratio and even your 'visceral fat' level, which is the fat around your vital organs. This is a strong indicator for health.

As you can imagine, all these statistics were of great interest to the group and they served as a great motivating factor as they set upon the Trial.

Fancy having a go yourself at the Fitness Test? You can find it in Chapter Ten, together with all the expected results for the different age groups from 60 years to 90 years.

7. The Exercise Trial

It was a real pleasure and a privilege to meet these volunteers, who were putting themselves forward into the unknown. I spent time getting to know them individually to discover their motivation for coming on the Trial. Even more important, was to find out what they were hoping to achieve as an end result. Unsurprisingly, most of the group said they wanted to drop a few pounds, but more encouragingly, the whole group were keen to find a suitable exercise programme appropriate to their age and to get started.

As part of the assessment process they were all officially measured for their height using a Stadiometer and almost without exception, they were all surprised when told their correct height. Because your height affects your Body Mass Index (BMI) calculation, it is important that we get this measurement accurately. If they had checked their BMI on an official website and put in the wrong height, they would have been given the wrong BMI reading. Sadly, it is a fact that inevitably, as we age, we are likely to lose some height, but it was quite amusing that one of the gentlemen was actually 3 inches shorter than he thought! His wife declared that she had never believed he was the height he had said he was from when they first met!

The average loss of height is between 1–2 inches (2–5cm), largely caused by the thinning of our cartilage between the vertebrae as we get older, but there's hope! It is really important to be aware that maintaining a good posture and exercising regularly can make a *big* difference to this and can help us to stem the decline.

Once all the tests were completed, it was very clear that although many were reasonably active with regular walking, e.g. to the shops, almost without exception they did not have adequate *strength* in either their upper or lower body, with poor *flexibility*, and none had ever tested their ability to *balance* on one leg. They were setting off to put that right.

Test Results

Marjory (age 69)

Marjory is one of those people you warm to instantly and she was SO keen to get going and to do everything right – an attitude that I love.

It is not uncommon to develop what is called a kyphotic spine as we get older, where our upper back has a curvature that makes our posture position less than perfect. Marjory had this condition, which meant that her forward head position put the weight of her head too far forward, putting a lot of pressure on the muscles in her neck and causing her balance to be seriously affected. But there is good news. I explained to Marjory that when someone with this condition is encouraged to lift to a better posture, they can make significant improvements. Ideally, when out walking she needs to concentrate on being as upright as possible, watching the ground by lowering her eyeline rather than leaning forward with the head and shoulders. Marjory was keen to try and decided to give herself regular reminders, so that she could make a real effort and hopefully see significant improvement with it. And that is what this Trial is all about – trying to improve what has become our norm over time, and training our body to be stronger and fitter going forward. I welcomed the challenge that Marjory presented and I could not have had a more willing and enthusiastic student!

Marjory's initial fitness test was not good. She was below average in all of the strength tests and 'poor' on the balance test. We both realised there was work to be done.

Here are Marjory's results after 28 days: Her **Lower Body Strength** had gone from 'below average' to 'excellent', as did her **Upper Body Flexibility**. In total, Marjory had improved significantly in five categories of the test, which is remarkable in such a short time – including her ability to balance.

After the final assessment, Marjory said: 'I feel so much fitter! I am walking faster and I'm so pleased with all my results in just four weeks. I have a problem with balance so I do struggle with that, but I'm determined to improve it even more with regular practice. The exercises in the Plan are achievable and I am determined to continue to exercise on a regular basis. Based on my experience, I would strongly recommend this plan to others.'

During the month of the Trial, Marjory had lost 6.5lbs, which was great, and her BMI had dropped from 27.6 to 26.4 – very close to the 'healthy' level of 25. What surprised Marjory most was that her body fat had dropped from 32.3 per cent to 28.3 per cent – in just four weeks!

Peter (age 75) and Jenny (age 74)

Peter and his wife Jenny joined the Trial and initially it felt a bit like his wife was the driving force and he was joining in, perhaps to encourage her to do more exercise. Unfortunately, Jenny had a foot problem during the Trial, which limited her from completing the programme and she was unable to participate in the final fitness test. However, Peter took up the mantle and made some significant improvements to his health over the 28 days.

Peter has been on medication for high blood pressure for over 30 years and had bowel cancer 12 years ago, for which, thankfully, he has been given the all clear. Peter acknowledged that he was very overweight and at the start of the Trial I weighed him on the Tanita Body Composition Scales. He weighed in with a BMI of 29, and unfortunately had a high visceral fat reading (that's the fat that lies around your vital organs, putting him at greater risk of a stroke).

Peter approached the challenge enthusiastically and saw it as an opportunity to make a difference to his health. After the Trial, this is what he said: 'I feel considerably better for losing the weight and I'm surprised and delighted that my visceral fat level is reducing. This has been a real wake-up call for me. I thought I was fitter at the start of the Trial than the fitness test showed, but I will carry on with the exercises at my local gym. I've enjoyed it.'

The good news is that Peter improved significantly in two categories of the test: his **Upper Body Strength** and on the **Step Test**, attaining the 'excellent' category in both. He lost 6lbs and went from 29.3 per cent to 25.4 per cent body fat. Most importantly, his visceral fat reading dropped by almost 10 per cent – in just four weeks!

Despite Jenny not being able to finish the full fitness test, she still participated in two categories: **Upper Body Strength** and **Upper Body Flexibility**. She improved greatly in both areas, which showed she had been applying herself to the programme as much as she could. Her **Upper Body Strength** increased from 'below average' to 'above average', a significant improvement, and her **Upper Body Flexibility** increased by 10 per cent. It was disappointing for Jenny that she could not be tested on her stamina, as this was the area of fitness she felt she had put the most effort into.

Jenny said: 'With this Trial I really wanted to "kickstart" myself into a regular walking pattern and I have now proved to myself that a daily walk can be achieved, despite leading a busy life. I started at 30 minutes but eventually progressed to over an hour and despite not being able to do the leg strength retest, I know my legs are stronger and I have more energy. I was frustrated at not being able to complete the Trial but without doubt I will have another go!'

Jan (age 69)

When I first spoke with Jan I was concerned about her general health. Jan has multiple health problems, mostly linked to her severe arthritis, and there were concerns around her ability to take up an exercise programme despite the gentle start of the Week 1 plan. However, upon meeting Jan and being impressed with her positive attitude, and after checking she could cope with all the exercises in Week 1, she embarked on the programme with great intentions.

Jan was surprised and delighted with her achievement and this is what she said: 'I managed to walk 20–30 minutes a day and if I couldn't go out, I would walk on the spot at home for 20 minutes! I certainly don't ache as much as I used to around my hips. Because of the various mobility issues I face, I know that I need to continue with the exercise myself as it has definitely had a positive effect on my daily life. I was surprised and pleased with the results – particularly my weight loss. I feel so much better in myself and I have more energy and enthusiasm for doing things. I would definitely recommend this Plan, particularly for others with mobility problems like mine.'

Jan stuck to the Plan to the letter and never faltered and, unsurprisingly, great things happened. She lost a stone and after I retested Jan at the end of the four weeks, she had improved her scores in an amazing four categories, making her a star student. The most significant change was in her walking, moving from the 'below average' category in Week 1 to the 'excellent' category four weeks later – remarkable!

Chris (age 76)

Chris was quite fit when she entered the programme and enjoys a group exercise session locally. Whilst not very overweight, she was looking for inspiration to lose a few pounds and to do extra regular exercise, particularly more walking. Chris is clearly a keen advocate of staying fit and was one of my older trialists. Chris's great enthusiasm as she embarked on the exercise programme was impressive – and it paid off!

After the final test Chris said: 'I am so glad I took part in this Trial. I have lost weight, have more energy and feel a definite improvement in my digestive system, which is a real bonus. I am very pleased that my fitness improved to the extent that it did *and* that I lost 6lbs in weight! I just loved the walking and found it not only good for the body but also for the soul. It is so important in my age group to stay fit and well and I would encourage others to give it a go – it definitely worked for me.'

Despite being quite fit already, in the 28 days Chris moved up a category in four areas of the fitness test and in the **Step Test** she went way beyond 'excellent'! She made significant improvements in her stamina, strength and flexibility, demonstrating that she had stuck to the programme religiously. The great bonus was that Chris went from BMI 26.7 to 25.5 and almost into the 'healthy' range. A really impressive effort all round.

Ann (age 66)

Ann entered the Trial feeling very unfit and overweight. She has been fit in the past and really wanted to get that back and came into the Trial with considerable enthusiasm and great determination. It paid off.

Ann said: 'I wanted this to be a lifestyle change that

is with me for ever and not just a "diet". I want all-round better health. Every year I pick up every winter bug going and I want that to be different, particularly with COVID-19 around.

'I felt it was easy to commit to the level of exercise required on this Plan – if it had been too vigorous or too time consuming, it would have put me off.

'My upper body was very weak and I feel that it has now improved immensely and I have also felt the benefit of the tummy exercises. I honestly feel much better and less sluggish and my clothes look a lot better on me. Would I recommend this programme to others? Absolutely, without doubt – yes!! I already have and I feel very privileged to have been on the Trial.'

When I did the final test with Ann, she had improved in every element of the fitness test and had elevated her strength and stamina to 'excellent' in four categories! Ann was also delighted to have lost 5lbs in weight. She was a joy to work with and a pleasure to have on the Trial.

Roger (age 73) and Lyn (age 72)

This lovely couple came on to the Trial with all good intentions and wanting to do their very best to stay healthy in their later years. Roger has been diagnosed with Alzheimer's and you could tell immediately how Lyn was keen to keep Roger as fit as possible despite the life-changing diagnosis. They are a well-travelled couple and keen to keep life going as normal as possible. Lyn came into the Trial fairly fit despite having a BMI of 28.8. She did lose a few pounds, dropping her BMI a little, but her best result was in the fitness test where she improved by 10 per cent in all areas, and particularly her **Upper Body Flexibility** improved from 'below average' to 'above average', which showed an improvement in her posture.

Due to Roger's condition, he found it difficult to give feedback on the Trial, but Lyn spoke for both of them by saying, 'The timing of the Trial proved to be rather difficult as we were having renovations to the kitchen, which turned out to be rather stressful. We did manage though to get out for walks and my legs certainly feel stronger for it and we hope to follow up the Trial with more commitment when the building work is complete. The body composition on the Tanita scales was very enlightening as I have lost some height and appreciated being given a professional assessment of our BMI and body fat levels, which was very useful.'

Jen (age 61)

Jen turned out to be one of my neighbours whom I had never met before, but she saw the posting on the 'Next Door' App, the neighbours forum, where I had posted my details of the Trial, and she was keen to join. My posting attracted great attention as I think most postings are for neighbours looking for a plumber! Jen was quite fit already because she was a regular walker, so her legs were fit and strong. However, it is important that we all exercise our total body so that our mid and upper body are also strong. Jen set out to put that right as these were areas that didn't benefit from walking.

Despite a shoulder injury that restricted her progressing

her press-ups at the wall to the floor, she managed to increase her **Upper Body Strength** from 'below average' to 'above average', which was great. Her injury also improved so much that her **Upper Body Flexibility** progressed from 'below average' to 'excellent', which showed that taking a whole-body approach to fitness can really pay off in such a short time. Jen was also keen to lose some weight, starting at BMI 27.7 and dropping to 26.5 by losing 6lbs, which really pleased her. Jen said, 'I feel far more positive about myself and much fitter all round. I found four weeks to be an ideal time frame, rapidly seeing benefits but not so long to risk losing motivation. I want to continue following the same regime as I have enjoyed seeing and feeling the benefits. My husband also lost weight and I have already recommended the programme to my sisters and a friend.'

Mark (age 69)

Unfortunately, on the first week of the Trial, Mark and his wife were away in Salcombe but because Mark was so keen to be included, I agreed to let him start a week later. Upon his return from holiday he attacked the programme with fantastic determination.

Mark entered this programme with all guns firing! His enthusiasm was a pleasure to work with and judging by the detailed food diary that he presented, he had made a real effort.

Mark is bipolar and therefore suffers significant mood swings and it was hoped that getting fitter and healthier may help to reduce the severity of these. His wife is an amazing support to him and they both embarked on the challenges of the Trial with equal gusto!

At the end of the Trial Mark had lost an amazing 10lbs and then there was the exercise side, where Mark also did really well. In all areas he improved his scores by 10 per cent or more. The biggest improvement was in his **Flexibility**, which is an area of fitness he had never focused on before, moving from 'poor' to 'average'. But now Mark adds stretching after every walk and strength workout. This will enable him to have greater mobility around his joints and, inevitably, everyday jobs will become easier.

Mark commented, 'I was really surprised with most of my readings from the body composition assessment. I thought I was a lot taller for a start, and my fat percentage is too high, so I need to carry on with this way of eating and exercising. I have achieved more than I thought I could and I am delighted with the results. Mentally I find it a struggle, but I know I need to keep at it!'

Alva (age 69)

When Alva joined the Trial team, she acknowledged that she was very overweight and realised she was putting her health at risk. The opportunity to volunteer was just the push she needed to do something about it. She knew that if she didn't take action, alarm bells would be ringing for her future health.

Alva also suffered from severe arthritis and had already had a knee replacement. This might have deterred Alva from starting a regular exercise programme but that was certainly not the case. In all elements of the fitness test

Alva made enormous improvements, going from 'below average' in five of the six tests to 'excellent' in three of them! I thought this was quite remarkable and clearly demonstrated just how much effort she had put into it!

Alva knew though that there was still a lot of work to do to come into the safe levels with her weight and body fat. She said, 'Before I was retested, I knew I had lost 7lbs but I had an indulgent weekend which skewed my end result on the scales. Despite all that, I do feel so much better. Walking is much easier and faster and I am leaving my friends behind! I am much more mentally alert and am completing tasks that would have daunted me before. I am *so* grateful for this Trial as I have learnt that I *can* follow an exercise plan aimed at my age group.'

Anne (age 63)

Anne came into this programme at a healthy BMI of 23.3 and with a good level of fitness. I was interested in her joining us because she was very keen to improve the health of her gut and was concerned that it was having a detrimental effect on her immune system. She feels she has a 'sluggish system' and regularly has to take laxatives to stay regular. A colonoscopy had revealed polyps, which can cause problems in the future. Her desire to improve this was very strong and very commendable.

Even with the first test she scored in the 'excellent' category with all except **Upper Body Strength**, which she managed to pull up to average over the 28 days. She lost weight, which brought her to what is termed **optimum**

BMI of 22.4 (halfway through the healthy range of 20–25), which was absolutely brilliant.

Anne commented, 'I am now fitter and more toned and my upper body strength has really improved, which I am very happy about. I am sleeping better and am more disciplined about what I will eat and when I will exercise. I now walk with much more purpose! I would recommend this programme as it gives you a great kickstart and is very easy to follow.'

I was delighted to hear from Ann a week after the final retest appointment with a text saying she was now definitely feeling some benefit in her gut – clearly in Anne's case it took just a bit longer than the 28 days for such improvements to show. Another very good reason to keep it up in the long term!

I was fascinated by the results of my trialist group as some of them presented with some complex health issues, which can be typical in many older people. I was so impressed with their determination and efforts to do the very best they could and their overall results were very positive and really encouraging. If they continue on the Plan, as Rosemary's trialists did, they will undoubtedly experience significant ongoing improvement.

Test yourself!

There is nothing more exciting than measuring our progress when we take on a challenge. All the tests that our trialists underwent are set out in Chapter Ten and it would be a really good idea to try them out for yourself to discover your current fitness level, according to your age group, before you start The 28-Day Immunity Plan. You can record your scores on the Fitness Test Progress Chart at the end of the book.

The instructions are set out for each test and then the norms are listed, so you can tell at a glance which category you fall into at the start. You can then assess which areas need more attention during the 28-day Plan in order to hopefully reach an appropriate level for your age.

Even if you are under the age of 60, you can still complete these tests. By following the exercise plan in this book regularly over the 28 days you will be amazed at the transformation in your fitness in just four weeks. The body is remarkably responsive to regular exercise and you will be so encouraged to measure the difference and that will, in turn, motivate you to continue going forward.

Not only is it important to undertake these tests with another person, it is much more fun too. They can help you time the test with a stopwatch and be sure to measure with a ruler or tape measure where needed (you are not taking body measurements, so don't worry). 'Buddying-up' with another like-minded friend or spouse, testing each other and then following the Plan together will seriously increase your motivation!

8. The 28-Day Immunity-Boosting Workout

How to Use This Programme

There are just eight strengthening exercises that over the four weeks will become progressively more challenging and increasingly effective.

If the first week's programme is too gentle for you, increase the number of repetitions according to your level of fitness or begin with Week 2.

If the first week is too challenging for you, see how much you can do and try to progress your workout each day.

Ideally, the walking (Stamina Training) is to be done every day and the Strength Programme four times per week for best results.

Safety tips

- Never exercise if you feel unwell.
- Keep drinking water to stay well hydrated.
- Doing the walk, followed by the strength exercises, ensures that the body is warm before applying 'resistance' to strengthen your muscles.
- Wear loose and comfortable clothing with good walking shoes when walking outdoors and

comfortable trainers or similar when exercising
indoors.

- Always check with your doctor if you have any
underlying health issues or doubts about your
ability to undertake this or any other exercise
programme.

Week One: Gentle Start

Stamina Training

Walk for 15 minutes per day every day this week.

Calf Stretch and Front Thigh Stretch

- On completing every walk, stretch your calf
  muscles by standing, taking one foot in front of
  the other. Keep your back leg straight, feet
  parallel and bend the knee of your front leg. Feel
  the stretch in the calf of your back leg. Repeat
  with the other leg forward. Hold the stretch for
  6–8 seconds on each leg.

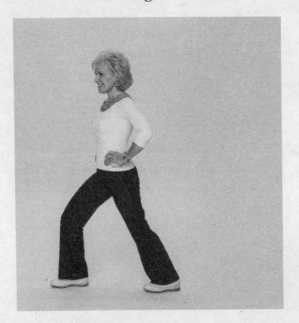

- To stretch your quads, bend your left leg and with your left hand take hold of your left ankle (or trouser leg) and bring the thighs close together in line with each other, then stand upright to stretch the front of your left thigh. Hold for 6–8 seconds, then change legs. Hold on to a chair for support if necessary.

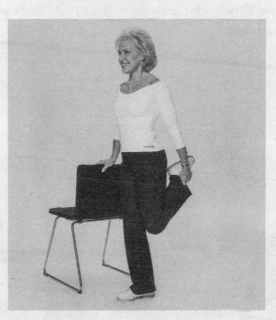

Strength Programme

Repeat this workout (exercises and stretches) 4 times a week.

Equipment: a sturdy dining chair and light weights, such as 2 x 500ml water bottles, tins of beans or 1kg hand weights

Exercise 1 Thigh Strengthener

Sit to stand: sit on a sturdy chair in the front third of the seat with feet flat on the floor, hip-width apart. Bring the feet back a little and lean forward slightly with arms by your side. Now, without using your hands to assist you, stand up in one swift movement, then lower back to the seat more slowly and gently return to the start position. Repeat 8 times.

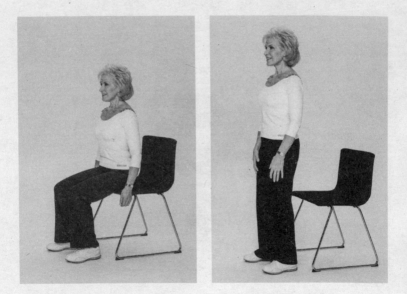

Exercise 2 Shoulder Strengthener

Stand upright with a weight in each hand and holding your core tight. Now, lift the weights out to the side, but only to shoulder height. Lower again under control. Keep the shoulders pulling down as the arms lift and make sure your arms are in your peripheral vision when at shoulder height. Repeat 8 times slowly.

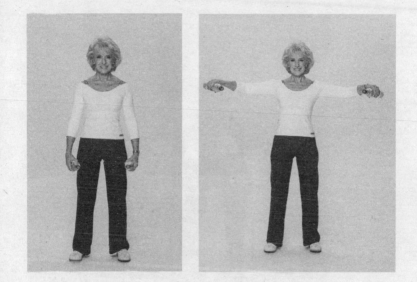

Exercise 3 Core Strengthener

Sit upright in the front third of the chair seat with a weight in each hand down by your sides. Pull the tummy in firmly and keep it held in tight as you bend to the side, allowing your hand weight to lower, keeping your spine from leaning forward or back. Lift back to the upright position, then bend to the other side. Do 12 repetitions (6 to each side).

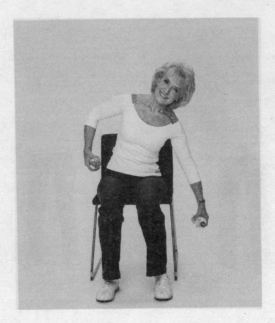

Exercise 4 Posture Improver

Sitting upright with a weight in each hand, hold them in front of you with elbows close to the waist (bent at a 90-degree angle) and palms up. Keeping the elbows close to the waist, separate the hands to take them out to the side, drawing the shoulder blades together behind you. Hold for a slow count of 2 and then release. Repeat 10 times slowly.

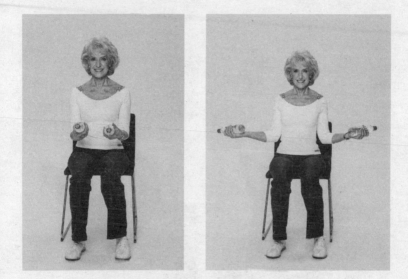

Exercise 5 Bone Strengthener

Stand behind the chair with hands on the top of the chair back. Now bend both knees in preparation to jump. With tummy held tight for support, jump with both feet only just leaving the floor and use the back of the chair to aid you. Land softly, bending the knees. If you hardly lift that is fine, but feel a solid landing onto the floor to strengthen your bones. Do 12 mini-jumps.

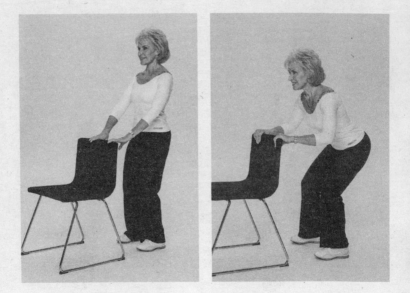

Exercise 6 Chest and Upper Body Strengthener

Wall press-ups: stand half a metre away from a clear wall. Place your hands flat on the wall, slightly wider than shoulder-width apart and at shoulder height. Holding the tummy in tight for support and keeping the body straight, bend the elbows, taking the forehead towards the wall. Push back, keeping the hands fully connected to the wall. Repeat 10 times slowly.

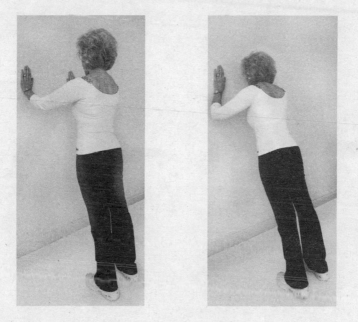

Holding on to the back of a chair with both feet parallel and hip-width apart, bend both knees and, as you straighten again, lift the right leg out to the side. Return to the middle and then lift the left leg out. Keep the body upright throughout. Repeat 16 times (8 each leg).

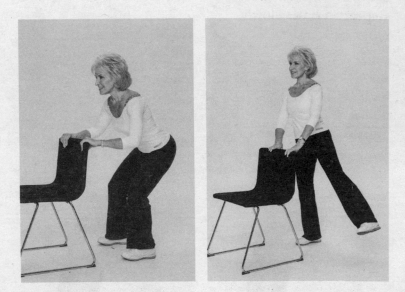

Exercise 8 Balance Trainer

With the chair ready for support if necessary, stand tall and in a good posture without shoes. Pull the tummy in and take one foot slowly off the floor to balance. If you start losing your balance, then touch the chair for support. Keep letting go, trying to reach 5 seconds without seeking support. Change legs and repeat. Focusing on a static object straight in front of you whilst you balance will help.

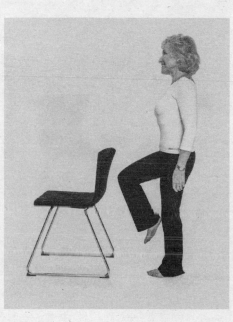

Stretches

Back Thigh Stretch

Sit on the edge of a chair seat and extend one leg out on the floor in line with the hip. Now, keeping the back straight and hands on your thighs, lean forward to feel a stretch at the back of that thigh. Pull the toes of that foot towards you and hold for 10 seconds. Change legs.

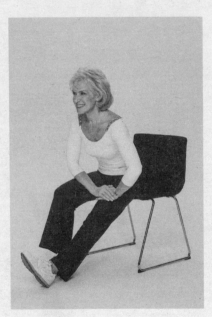

Posture Stretch

Sit upright and take both arms behind you, clasping the hands. Keeping the shoulders down, feel the shoulder blades drawn together behind you as you stretch your chest. Hold for 10 seconds.

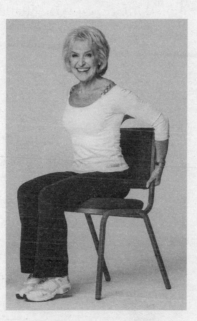

Front Thigh Stretch

Stand behind a chair, holding on with one hand for support. Now lift one foot off the floor and hold the ankle (or your sock or trouser leg). The thighs need to be together and the body upright. Hold for 10 seconds then change legs.

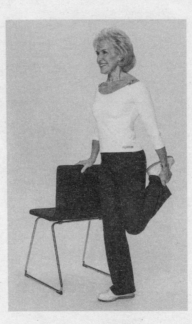

Week Two: Progressing Our Strength

Stamina Training

Walk for 20 minutes per day every day this week.

Calf Stretch and Front Thigh Stretch

- On completing every walk, stretch your calf muscles by standing, taking one foot in front of the other. Keep your back leg straight, feet parallel and bend the knee of your front leg. Feel the stretch in the calf of your back leg. Repeat with the other leg forward. Hold the stretch for 6–8 seconds on each leg.

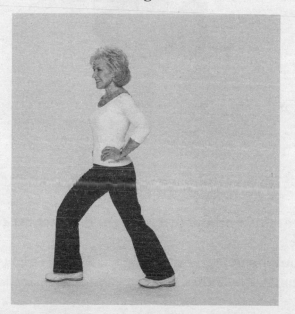

- To stretch your quads, bend your left leg and with your left hand take hold of your left ankle (or trouser leg) and bring the thighs close together in line with each other, then stand upright to stretch the front of your left thigh. Hold for 6–8 seconds, then change legs. Hold on for support if necessary.

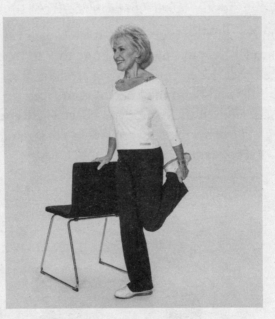

Strength Programme

Repeat this workout (exercises and stretches) 4 times a week.

Equipment: a sturdy dining chair, light weights, such as 500ml water bottles, tins of beans or 1kg hand weights and a small rolled-up towel to place under your head if you wish.

Note: if you are unable to exercise on the floor, try doing exercises 4, 5, 6 and 7 lying on your bed.

Exercise 1 Thigh Strengthener

Sit to stand: sit on a sturdy chair in the front third of the seat with feet flat on the floor, hip-width apart. Bring the feet back a little and lean forward slightly with arms by your side. Now, without using your hands to assist you, stand up in one swift movement, then lower back to the seat more slowly and gently return to the start position. Repeat 12 times.

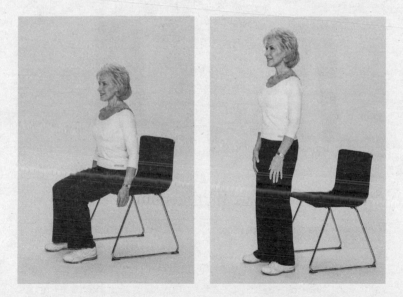

Exercise 2 Shoulder Strengthener

Stand upright with a weight in each hand and holding your core tight. Now, lift the weights out to the side, but only to shoulder height. Lower again under control. Keep the shoulders pulling down as the arms lift and make sure your arms are in your peripheral vision when at shoulder height. Repeat 8 times slowly. Rest and repeat another set.

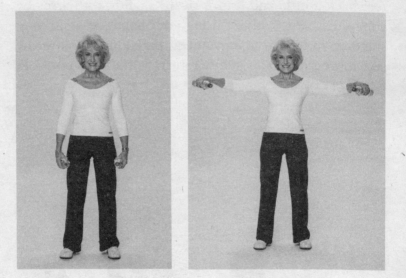

Stand behind the chair with hands on the top of the chair back. Now bend both knees in preparation to jump. With tummy held tight for support, jump with both feet only just leaving the floor and use the back of the chair to aid you. Land softly, bending the knees. If you hardly lift that is fine, but feel a solid landing onto the floor to strengthen your bones. Do 12 mini-jumps, rest and repeat.

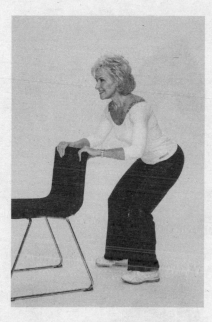

Exercise 4 Core Strengthener

Lie on your back with the towel under your head (optional). Place your hands behind your head. Then reach your left hand to the left thigh. Pull in the tummy and breathe in. As you breathe out, lift your head and shoulders off the floor and slide the left hand up towards the knee. Lower again under control. Do 8 repetitions. Change arms and repeat.

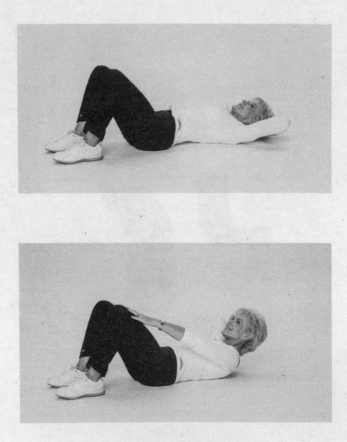

Exercise 5 Upper Body Strengthener

With hands and knees on the floor, place the hands directly under your shoulders and the knees under your hips. Pull in the tummy to support the back and bend the elbows as you lower the forehead towards the floor as you breathe in. Now as you breathe out, push up again, straightening the elbows without locking them out at the top. Do 6 repetitions, then sit back to rest. Then do another set of 6.

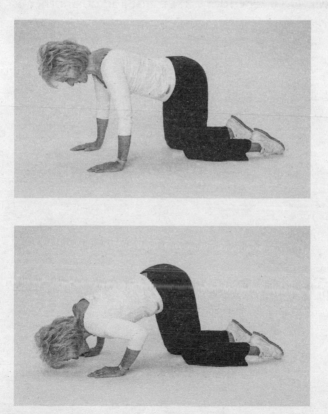

Exercise 6 Back Strengthener and Posture Improver

Lie on the floor on your front with your hands on the floor, elbows bent and palms facing upwards. Pull your tummy in to support the back and keep the legs hip-width apart and relaxed. Breathe in and as you breathe out, lift your head and shoulders whilst pulling your shoulders down away from your ears. Press the ribs at the front into the floor to feel the muscles of the mid-back working. Hold for a slow count of 2 and then breathe in as you lower. Do 6 repetitions, then rest and do another 6.

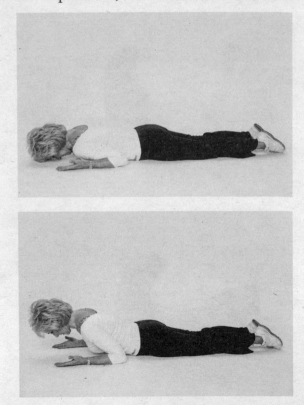

Exercise 7 Hip Strengthener

Lie on your side with your underneath leg slightly bent, but with the top leg straight and in line with the rest of the body. Rest your head on the underneath arm. With your upper hand, hold a bottle of water or small weight on top of your thigh to provide resistance. Pull the toes of the top leg toward you and turn the foot down slightly. Now lift the top leg, under control, making sure the hips stay stacked on top of each other, then lower. Lift and lower 12 times on each side and then repeat another set.

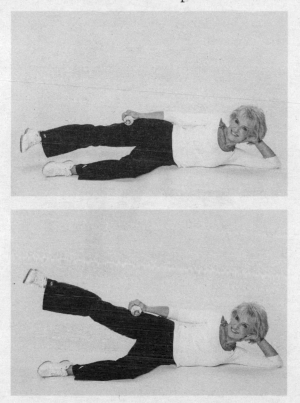

With the chair ready for support if necessary, stand tall and in a good posture without shoes. Pull the tummy in and take one foot slowly off the floor to balance. If you start losing your balance, then touch the chair for support. Keep letting go, trying to reach 10 seconds without seeking support. Change legs and repeat. Focusing on a static object straight in front of you whilst you balance will help.

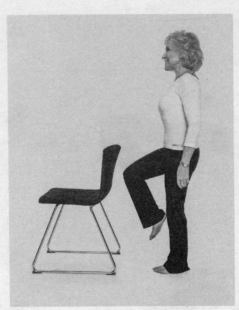

Stretches

Front Thigh Stretch

Lie on your front and place your right hand under your forehead. Bend the left leg, taking hold of the ankle (or trouser leg) with your left hand. Bring the knees together and press the left hip into the floor to feel the stretch at the front of the hip of the bent leg. Hold for 10 seconds, then repeat with the other leg.

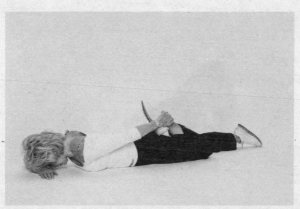

Hip and Back Thigh Stretch

Lie on your back with both knees bent and feet flat on the floor. Take hold behind the right leg. Now straighten that leg, keeping the hips firmly on the floor, holding the back of your thigh and calf with your hands to feel a stretch at the back of the right thigh. Hold for 10 seconds, then breathe in and, as you breathe out, try to straighten the right leg further. Hold for another 10 seconds, then bend it to return to the start position. Repeat the stretch with your left leg.

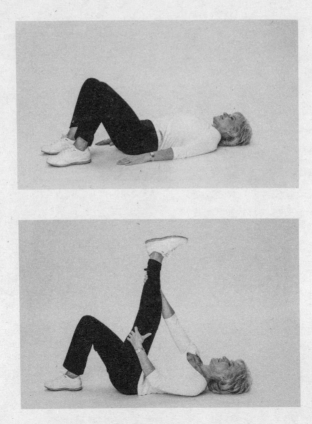

Posture Stretch

Stand upright and take both hands clasped behind your back. Keep the shoulders down and look straight ahead as you lift the arms up behind you to stretch across the chest. Hold for 10 seconds.

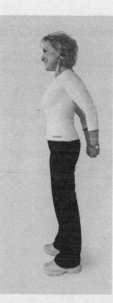

Week Three: Challenging and Strengthening

Stamina Training

Walk for 25 minutes per day every day this week and now try to walk with more purpose and intensity.

Calf Stretch and Front Thigh Stretch

- On completing every walk, stretch your calf muscles by standing, taking one foot in front of the other. Keep your back leg straight, feet parallel and bend the knee of your front leg. Feel the stretch in your calf of the back leg. Repeat with the other leg forward. Hold the stretch for 6–8 seconds on each leg.

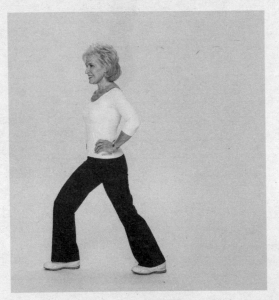

- To stretch your quads, bend your left leg and with your left hand take hold of your left ankle (or trouser leg) and bring the thighs close together in line with each other, then stand upright to stretch the front of your left thigh. Hold for 6–8 seconds, then change legs. Hold on for support if necessary.

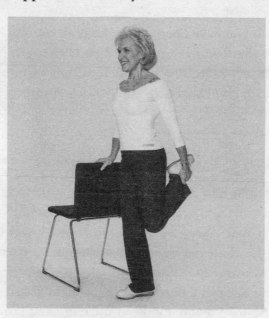

Strength Programme

Repeat this workout (exercises and stretches) 4 times a week.

Equipment: a sturdy dining chair, light weights, such as 2 x 500ml water bottles (or even try 2 x 1 litre bottles for greater resistance), or 2kg hand weights and a small rolled-up towel

Note: If you have been doing the floor exercises on the bed, now that you have increased your strength it would be good to try exercising on the floor, but with the aid of a chair seat close by to help you get down and up again if necessary.

Exercise 1 Thigh Strengthener

Stand upright half a step away from a sturdy chair with hands on your hips and tummy pulled in. Stand with feet hip-width apart. Now bend the knees and lower the hips close to the chair seat (without sitting on it), then lift up again slowly and smoothly. Try not to lock out the knees at the top. Keep the head looking straight ahead. Repeat 8 times. Sit for a few seconds on the chair and then repeat another set of 8.

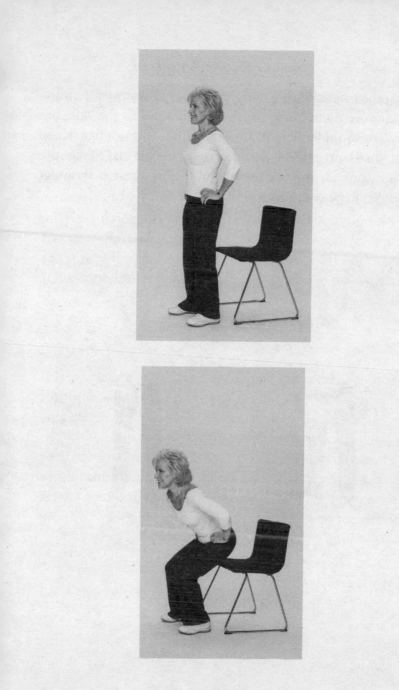

Stand upright with a weight in each hand and holding your core tight. Now, lift the weights out to the side, but only to shoulder height. Lower again under control. Keep the shoulders pulling down as the arms lift and make sure your arms are in your peripheral vision when at shoulder height. Repeat 10 times slowly. Rest and repeat.

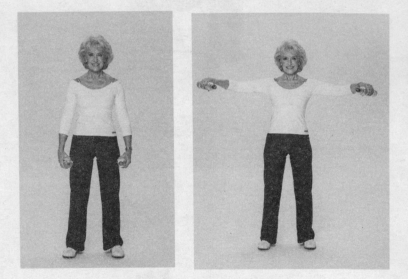

Standing tall and with tummy held in tightly, pretend to skip with both feet leaving the floor if possible, bending the knees as you land and ensuring your heels touch the floor. Imagine holding a skipping rope to help you with the rhythm. If you can only semi-skip that is fine, but landing firmly with your heels to the floor will stimulate your bones. Do 3 lots of 12 skips.

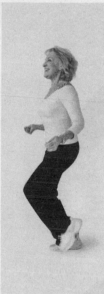

- Lie on your back with knees bent and feet hip-width apart. Place both hands behind your head. Pull the tummy in tight and breathe in then, as you take a slow out breath, lift your head and shoulders off the floor. Hold for a slow count of 2 and lower again with control. Feel the weight of the head in your hands to support the neck. Repeat 8 times.

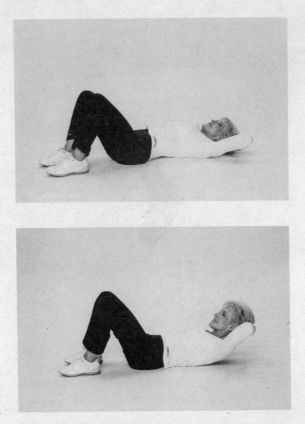

- To strengthen the muscles of the waist, remain lying on your back with your knees bent and with your hands behind your head. Lift your head and shoulders, but this time reach across with your right hand toward your left knee and hold for 2 counts, then slowly lower again. Lift and twist to the other knee with the other hand, hold for 2 counts, then lower again. Repeat 8 times (4 to each side). Rest and repeat.

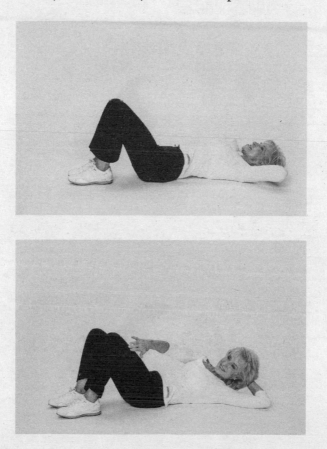

With hands and knees on the floor, place the hands directly under your shoulders and the knees further back. Pull in the tummy to support the back and bend the elbows as you lower the forehead towards the floor as you breathe in. Now as you breathe out, push up again, straightening the elbows without locking them out at the top. Do 10 repetitions, then sit back to rest. Then do another set of 10.

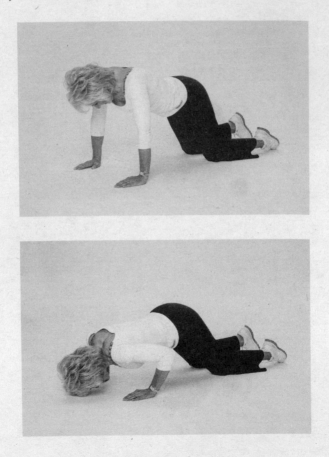

Exercise 6 Back Strengthener and Posture Improver

Lie on your front with your arms by your side and legs parallel. Place your forehead on a towel if you wish. Now breathe in, holding your core tight, and as you breathe out, lift the head whilst still looking at the floor. At the same time, lift the arms from the floor, turning palms to face the thighs, and squeeze your shoulder blades together. Hold this position for 2 seconds, then release down again. Do 8 repetitions.

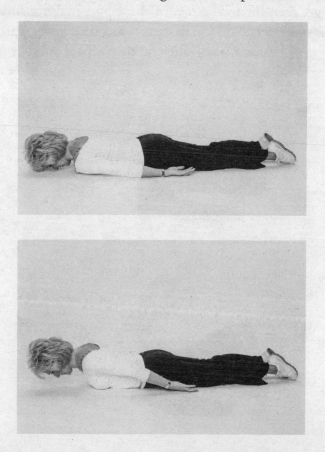

Lie on your side with your underneath leg slightly bent, but with the top leg straight and in line with the rest of the body. Rest your head on the underneath arm. With your upper hand, hold a bottle of water or small weight on top of your thigh to provide resistance. Pull the toes of the top leg toward you and turn the foot down slightly. Now lift the top leg, under control, stopping halfway through the range, then lift to the top of the range, making sure the hips stay stacked on top of each other, then lower. Lift and lower 16 times on each side and then repeat another set.

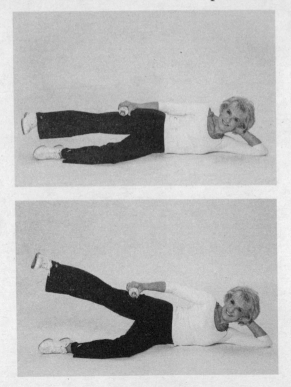

With the chair ready for support if necessary, stand tall and in a good posture without shoes. Pull the tummy in and take one foot slowly off the floor to balance. If you start losing your balance, then touch the chair for support. Keep letting go, trying to reach 20 seconds without seeking support. Change legs and repeat. Focusing on a static object straight in front of you whilst you balance will help.

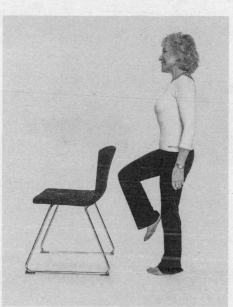

Stretches

Front Thigh Stretch

Lie on your front and bend one knee, taking hold of the ankle (or trouser leg). Bring the knees together and press the hip into the floor on the bent leg to feel the stretch at the front of that hip. Hold for 10 seconds, then change legs and repeat.

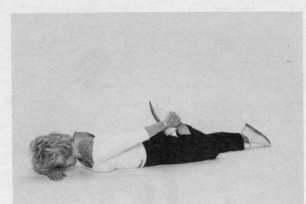

Hip and Back Thigh Stretch

Lie on your back with both knees bent and feet flat on the floor. Take hold behind the right leg. Now straighten that leg, keeping the hips firmly on the floor, holding the back of your thigh and calf with your hands to feel a stretch at the back of the right thigh. Hold for 10 seconds, then breathe in and, as you breathe out, try to straighten the right leg further. Hold for another 10 seconds, then bend it to return to the start position. Repeat the stretch with your left leg.

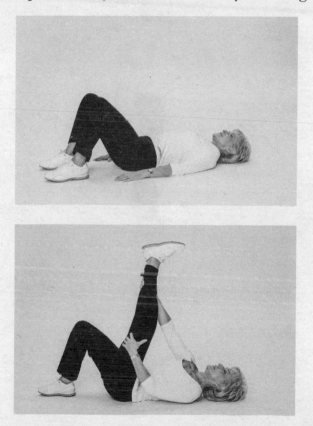

Posture Stretch

Stand upright and clasp both hands behind your back. Keep the shoulders down and look straight ahead as you lift the arms up behind you to stretch across the chest. Hold for 10 seconds.

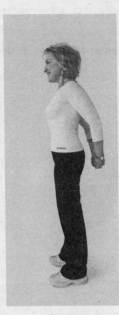

Week Four: Advanced Workout

Stamina Training

Walk for 30 minutes or more per day every day this week. Vary your route and try to add some inclines to challenge you more.

Calf Stretch and Front Thigh Stretch

- On completing every walk, stretch your calf muscles by standing, taking one foot in front of the other. Keep your back leg straight, feet parallel and bend the knee of your front leg. Feel the stretch in your calf of the back leg. Repeat with the other leg forward. Hold the stretch for 6–8 seconds on each leg.

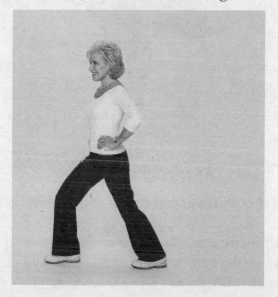

- To stretch your quads, bend your left leg and with your left hand take hold of your left ankle (or trouser leg) and bring the thighs close together in line with each other, then stand upright to stretch the front of your left thigh. Hold for 6–8 seconds, then change legs. Hold on to a chair for support if necessary.

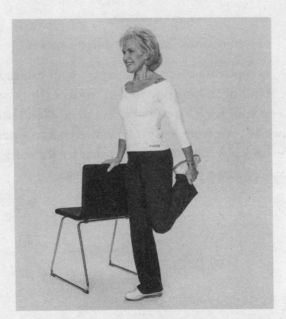

Strength Programme

Repeat this workout (exercises and stretches) 4 times a week.

Equipment: a sturdy dining chair, weights – progress to a max of 2kg hand weights or 2-litre bottles of water – and a small rolled-up towel

Note: If you have been doing the floor exercises on the bed, now that you have increased your strength it would be good to try exercising on the floor, but with the aid of a chair seat close by to help you get down and up again if necessary.

Exercise 1 Thigh Strengthener

Stand upright one step away from a sturdy chair with hands on your hips and tummy pulled in. Stand with feet hip-width apart. Now bend the knees and lower the hips close to the chair seat (without sitting on it), then lift up again slowly and smoothly. Try not to lock out the knees at the top. Keep the head looking straight ahead. Repeat 16 times in one go or split into 2 sets of 8.

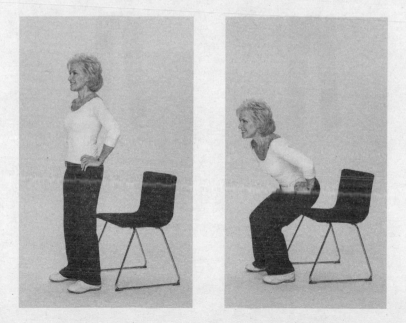

Stand upright with a weight in each hand and holding your core tight. Now lift the weights out to the side, but only to shoulder height. Lower again under control. Keep the shoulders pulling down as the arms lift and make sure your arms are in your peripheral vision when at shoulder height. Repeat 16 times slowly or split into 2 sets of 8.

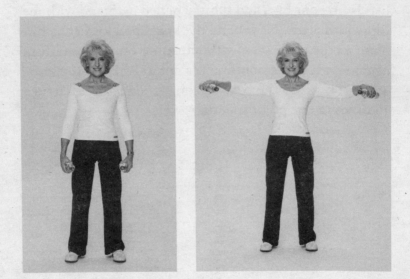

Exercise 3 Bone Strengthener

Standing with feet parallel, bend the knees and jump off the floor, landing fully through the feet with the heels touching the floor each time and with knees soft. Swing the arms in rhythm to give some momentum to the action. Alternatively, you can pretend skip on the spot, ensuring your heels land each time. Try to keep jumping rhythmically for 30 jumps or skips. This action works wonders in strengthening the bones.

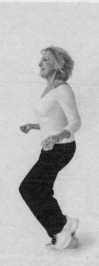

- Lie on your back with knees bent and feet hip-width apart. Place both hands behind your head. Pull the tummy in tight and breathe in then, as you take a slow out breath, lift your head and shoulders off the floor. Hold for a slow count of 4 and lower again with control. Feel the weight of the head in your hands to support the neck. Repeat 8 times.

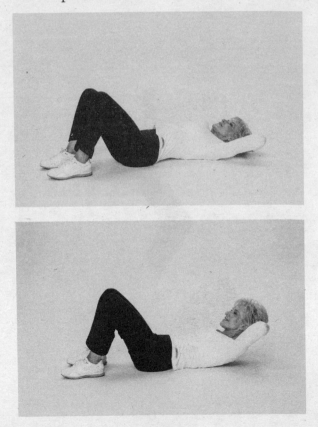

- To strengthen the muscles of the waist, remain lying on your back with your knees bent and with your hands behind your head. Lift your head and shoulders, but this time reach across with your right hand toward your left knee and hold for 2 counts, then slowly lower again. Lift and twist to the other knee with the other hand, hold for 2 counts, then lower again. Repeat 10 times (5 to each side).

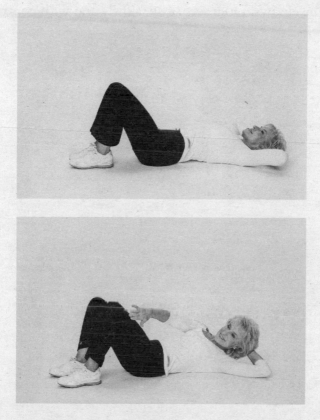

Rest and repeat both exercises.

Come up onto hands and knees on the floor with the hands directly under the shoulders, but now with the knees further back to suit your strength level. Holding your tummy in tightly throughout, lower the forehead towards the floor, slightly in front of the hands. Keep the head in line with the spine and keep your tummy pulled in to support your back. Push back up again without locking the elbows. Do 2 sets of 10, slowly and with control.

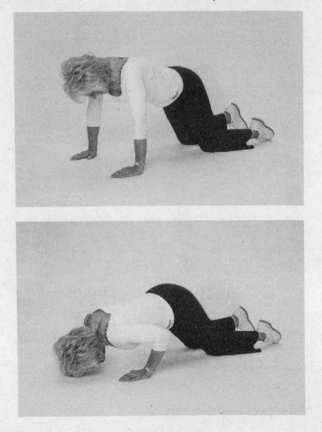

Lie on your front with the arms by your side and legs parallel. Place your forehead on a towel if you wish. Now breathe in, holding your core tight, and as you breathe out, lift the head whilst still looking at the floor. Hold this position for four seconds before releasing down. Try to keep shoulders pulled away from the ears. Do 8 repetitions. Rest and repeat.

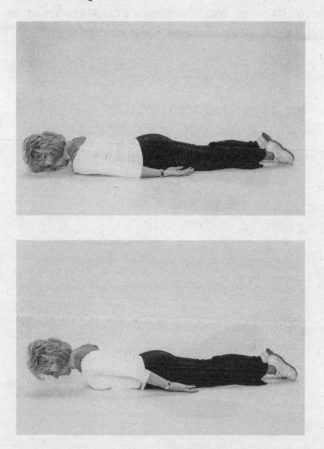

Lie on your side with your underneath leg slightly bent, but with the top leg straight and in line with the rest of the body. Rest your head on your hand of the underneath arm. With your upper hand, hold a bottle of water or small weight on top of your thigh to provide resistance. Pull the toes of the top leg toward you and turn the foot down slightly. Now lift the top leg, under control, with 3 separate stops to reach the top, and then lower in one movement. Repeat 10 times, then change legs.

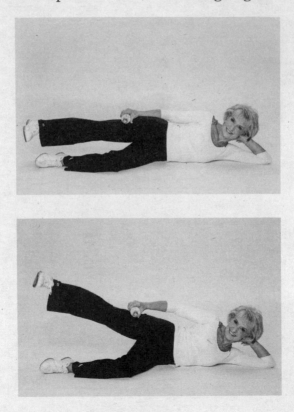

With the chair ready for support if necessary, stand tall
and in a good posture without shoes. Pull the tummy in
and take one foot slowly off the floor to balance. If you
start losing your balance, then touch the chair for support. Keep letting go, trying to reach a full 30 seconds
without seeking support. Change legs and repeat. Focusing on a static object straight in front of you whilst you
balance will help.

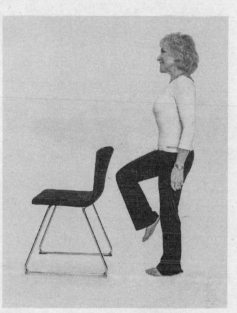

Stretches

Front Thigh Stretch

Lie on your front and place your right hand under your forehead. Bend the left leg, taking hold of the ankle (or trouser leg) with your left hand. Bring the knees together and press the left hip into the floor to feel the stretch at the front of the hip of the bent leg. Hold for 10 seconds, then repeat with the other leg.

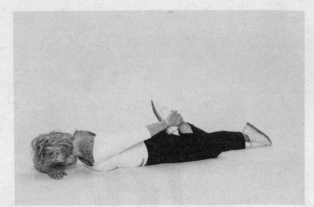

Hip and Back Thigh Stretch

Lie on your back with both knees bent and feet flat on the floor. Take hold behind the right leg. Now straighten that leg, keeping the hips firmly on the floor, holding the back of your thigh and calf with your hands to feel a stretch at the back of the right thigh. Hold for 10 seconds, then breathe in and, as you breathe out, try to straighten the right leg further. Hold for another 10 seconds, then bend it to return to the start position. Repeat the stretch with your left leg.

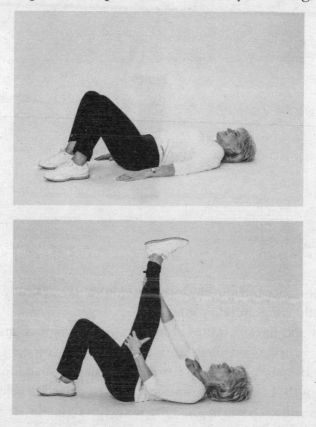

Stand upright and take both hands clasped behind your back. Keep the shoulders down and look straight ahead as you lift the arms up behind you to stretch across the chest. Hold for 10 seconds.

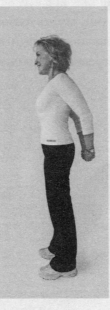

If you have completed this workout programme you should congratulate yourself.

If you haven't quite mastered all the progressions yet, keep working on them until you do. Once you get there, spend just 15 minutes, 3 times a week, to maintain the strength, balance and stamina that you have developed. This will keep you in great shape and give you the strength to live a much safer and more independent life into the future.

Continue with the daily walks for 30 minutes a day – this will keep your heart and lungs in great order and it will boost your immune system – and continue with the Strength Programme on 3 to 4 days each week to keep you strong. Enjoy being fitter.

9. Moving on to Greater Fitness

If you have mastered the previous programme and feel that you want to progress still further, here is a more advanced programme.

Stamina Training

If, after 28 days you can comfortably walk at a brisk pace and can include some inclines, then you might be ready for more of an aerobic challenge. You can move on to something called *slow jogging*, which is perfect for increasing the intensity of your Stamina Training but is actually performed at the same speed as walking. If you have concerns about your knees, hips and lower back, then it may not suit you, but if that is not the case, then certainly give it a go.

Benefits of Slow Jogging

- Pushes the cardiovascular system to the next level.
- Increases impact in a gentle way, strengthening bones.
- Burns calories at a faster rate, increasing rate of weight loss.
- Gives an extra boost to your immune system.

- Adopt the same speed at which you walk.
- Forget planting the heel first but place the whole foot down at the same time.
- Make the steps short and land softly.
- Keep your head up, watching the road ahead.
- You should be able to comfortably talk as you slow jog.
- Start with intervals of walk/slow jog – 1 minute on: 30 seconds off.

Stretches

Always do the Calf Stretch and Front Thigh Stretch after each session.

Calf Stretch and Front Thigh Stretch

- On completing every walk, stretch your calf muscles by standing, taking one foot in front of the other. Keep your back leg straight, feet parallel and bend the knee of your front leg. Feel the stretch in your calf of the back leg. Repeat with the other leg forward. Hold the stretch for 6–8 seconds on each leg.

- To stretch your quads, bend your left leg and with your left hand take hold of your left ankle (or trouser leg) and bring the thighs close together in line with each other, then stand upright to stretch the front of your left thigh. Hold for 6–8 seconds, then change legs. Hold on to a chair for support if necessary.

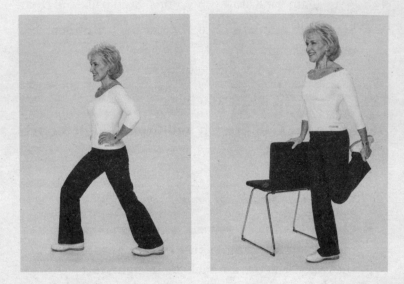

Enhanced Strength Programme

Exercise 1 Lunges

Stand tall with tummy in tight and take a large step forward with the right leg. Now keeping the trunk upright, bend both knees into a lunge with the front knee in line with the ankle. Straighten both legs, then bend and straighten again for 8 slow repetitions. Step back and then repeat with the other leg. Repeat 2 sets of 8 with each leg.

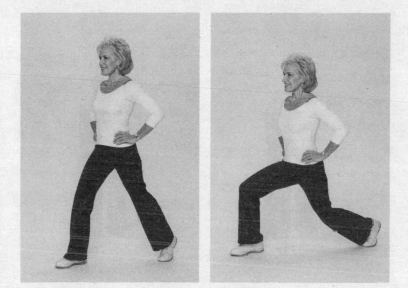

Stand tall with back straight, tummy held in and holding 1.5–2kg hand weights. Bring both arms up to shoulder height, keeping the shoulders down and relaxed. Now pull the left elbow back, bending the arm and keeping it at shoulder height. Turn the head to follow the elbow and keep the hips facing front. Do 8 repetitions to the same side, then change sides and repeat.

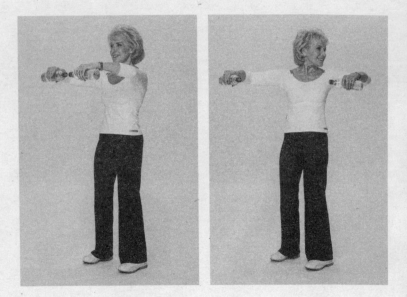

Lie on your front and lift onto forearms and knees, with toes curled under. Now breathe in and as you breathe out, pull tummy in very tight and lift the knees off the floor so your body forms a straight line from the top of your head to your feet. Breathe normally as you hold for 10 seconds, then release. Do 4 repetitions.

Adaptation: Keep both knees on the floor if needed.

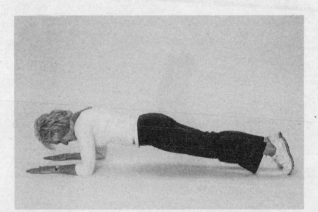

Exercise 4 *Advanced Waist Shaper*

Lie on your back with legs raised and ankles crossed. Place both hands behind the head with tummy in tight. Now breathe out as you lift head and shoulders off the floor. Hold this position as you reach the right hand up towards the left ankle, lifting the torso higher. Drop down slightly before reaching up again to the other side. Do 8 repetitions, then rest and repeat another set.

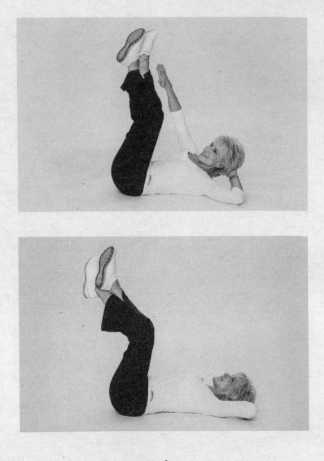

Exercise 5 Elongated Press-Up or Full Press-Up

Start on hands and knees with hands under the shoulders and your knees under the hips, then move your knees further back (or lift fully off the ground), pulling the tummy in tight. Breathe in as you lower the upper body towards the floor, bending elbows outwards and leading with the chest. Breathe out as you push back up again, without locking the elbows. Do 6 repetitions and build up to another set.

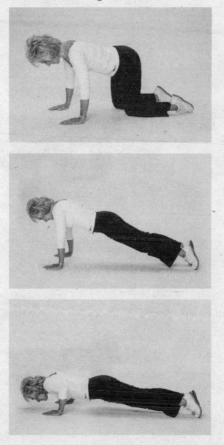

On hands and knees with shoulders in line with wrist and hips in line with knees, slide the right hand and left foot along the floor until leg and arm are as straight as possible. Hold tummy in as you lift the leg and arm off the floor in line with the trunk. Hold for a slow count of 3 and then release and repeat on the other side. Do 8 repetitions, changing sides each time.

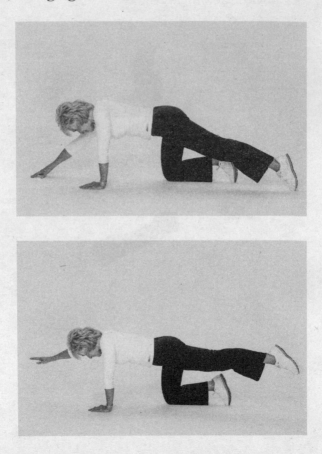

Stretches

Front Thigh Stretch

Lie on your front and place your right hand under your forehead. Bend the left leg, taking hold of the ankle (or trouser leg) with your left hand. Bring the knees together and press the left hip into the floor to feel the stretch at the front of the hip of the bent leg. Hold for 10 seconds, then repeat with the other leg.

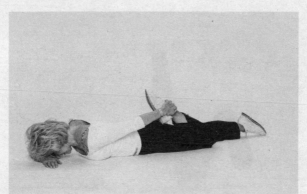

Hip and Back Thigh Stretch

Lie on your back with both knees bent and feet flat on the floor. Take hold behind the right leg. Now straighten that leg, keeping the hips firmly on the floor, holding the back of your thigh and calf with your hands to feel a stretch at the back of the right thigh. Hold for 10 seconds, then breathe in and, as you breathe out, try to straighten the right leg further. Hold for another 10 seconds, then bend it to return to the start position. Repeat the stretch with your left leg.

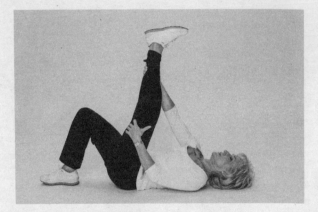

Posture Stretch

Sit upright with legs crossed and place both hands behind you on the floor. Keeping the shoulders down, draw the shoulders back to feel a stretch across the chest. Hold for 10 seconds.

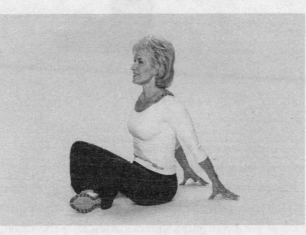

Back Stretch

Come up onto hands and knees and as you pull your tummy in, arch the spine up towards the ceiling, letting the head and neck hang loose. Hold for 6 seconds, then release.

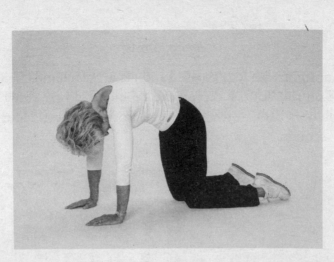

Lying Waist Stretch

Lie on your back with knees bent and together, feet flat on floor. Place arms out to the side at shoulder height with palms down. Pull tummy in and gently roll knees to the right side as you look at your left hand to feel a stretch in the waist. Hold for 6 seconds, then roll over to repeat on the other side.

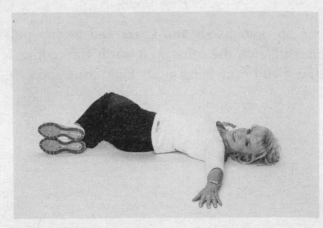

Full Body Stretch

Lie on your back with legs straight and take arms overhead. Stretch arms away from legs without arching the back. Hold for 6 seconds, then slowly release.

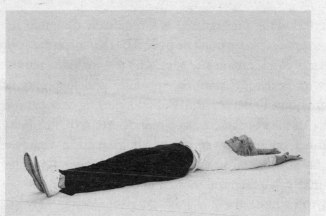

10. How to Do Your Own Fitness Test

The following programme is a medically designed test for the over 60s (please don't be put off by that if you are younger, as it is still relevant at any age). The test includes activities to measure strength, stamina, mobility and flexibility of the entire body. Different lifestyles and varying occupations can cause us to either gain or lose muscle strength, flexibility and stamina, but regular exercise can help us all, at whatever age, to stay strong and fit and live a fuller, longer, healthier and ultimately happier and more independent life.

In this book there is a 28-day progressive exercise plan suitable for all ages and abilities. By taking the test in this chapter *before* you start, or early on in the 28-day Plan, you will be able to see how much you have progressed by the end of the four-week programme and, hopefully, you will be so encouraged by your improvement that you will want to continue way beyond the four weeks – perhaps for the rest of your life.

You will need some basic equipment to be able to measure your fitness and flexibility, and a buddy to help you. Details of these are given at the top of each exercise. After each exercise you will see a chart organised into different age categories, giving the numbers of repetitions that are considered as being 'needs practice' to 'excellent'. Please make a note of your personal results on the Fitness Test Progress Chart on page 287.

Test 1

Lower Body Strength

Having enough strength in our legs is our number one priority. Without the ability to get up out of a chair, for example, and to be able to walk regularly throughout the day, the rest of the body will unfortunately go into serious decline. This is because the circulatory system will become sluggish, our lungs will be less challenged and the inevitable muscle wastage that follows would make us more susceptible to instability, illness and disease. *Leg strength* also helps reduce bone loss, maintain lean muscle tissue, prevent obesity (because we can move around more) and reduce the risk of falls. So, there are obviously a host of reasons why we should make the effort to do our weekly Strength Programme.

Lower Body Strength Test

Equipment: a sturdy dining chair and stopwatch (on your phone or use your watch)

- Sit in the middle of the chair seat with feet flat on the floor and slightly further back than normal, with arms across your chest.
- On the signal 'go', stand up to a full stand, then return to the fully seated position (it is important to avoid just touching the chair seat with the bottom), then stand up again.
- The score is the number of stand-ups and sit downs completed in 30 seconds.

Age Group	60+ F	M	70+ F	M	80+ F	M	90+ F	M
Excellent	17+	19+	15+	17+	14+	15+	11+	12+
Above Average	16	17	14	16	12	13	9	11
Average	14	16	12	14	11	12	7	9
Below Average	12	14	11	12	9	10	5	8
Needs Practice	10	12	9	10	7	8	3	6

Test 2

Upper Body Strength

Having a strong upper body is crucial to our independence. A good and well-maintained upper body strength is also vital for us to be able to carry out normal everyday functions, such as carrying shopping, lifting and moving objects and getting up from the floor. This would be particularly important if we were to have a fall so that we can get up again. The floor is also where grandchildren like to play and it is great if we can get down and join them.

Upper Body Strength Test

Equipment: 2.5kg hand weight (ladies) or a 4kg weight (men) If you don't have access to weights, then look for alternative options such as a shopping bag with two 1kg packs of rice or sugar plus a 500g pack/can of something, or even a hefty book or weighted door stop, which you can weigh on your bathroom scales.

You will also need a sturdy dining chair and a stopwatch

- Sit upright in the chair with feet flat on the floor.

- Hold the weight down by your side with your preferred arm straight toward the floor.
- On the signal 'go', bend your elbow and lift the weight up towards the shoulder. With each repetition go through the full range of movement. Try to avoid using momentum by keeping the upper arm still throughout the test.
- The score is the number of arm-curl weight-lifts completed in 30 seconds.

Age Group	60+ F	M	70+ F	M	80+ F	M	90+ F	M
Excellent	19+	22+	17+	21+	16+	19+	13+	14+
Above Average	17	20	16	19	14	17	12	13
Average	16	18	14	17	12	15	10	12
Below Average	14	17	12	15	11	14	9	10
Needs Practice	11	14	10	12	9	12	7	8

Test 3

Stamina

Stamina is critical for us to live an active and happy life. We usually know when we lack stamina as we feel generally lethargic and lack enough energy to carry out even the most menial tasks. The important thing to know is that we can *all*, at any age, increase our stamina dramatically. By starting slowly and gradually increasing our activity, we can truly make an enormous difference in a relatively short period of time. Almost without exception our trialists commented on their increased energy, and instead of the activity making them tired it was energising them. Stamina is all about how much oxygen we can take in through our lungs for us to use and this is called our 'aerobic capacity'. Unfortunately, our aerobic capacity declines with age (it can be as much as 50 per cent less by the age of 70), but don't despair. Studies indicate that *at least* half of this decline can be avoided simply by being physically active.

2-minute Step Test

Equipment: a stopwatch

- Stand upright in a clear space (as there is a tendency to move forward with this test).
- Lift one knee up to about halfway towards your hip (a 45 degree angle is about right).
- On the word 'go', begin stepping on the spot, bringing each knee to the correct height.
- The score is the number of full steps completed in 2 minutes, counted each time the right knee is lifted (i.e. alternate steps).

Age Group	60+ F	M	70+ F	M	80+ F	M	90+ F	M
Excellent	105+	115+	100+	110+	90+	100+	70+	85+
Above Average	95	105	90	100	80	90	65	80
Average	90	100	80	90	70	85	55	65
Below Average	80	90	70	85	65	75	50	55
Needs Practice	75	80	60	70	50	60	35	45

Test 4

Lower and Upper Body Flexibility

Flexibility is critical to everyday living. Lack of flexibility both in the lower and upper body can have serious consequences to how efficiently we move. It is often referred to as our 'range of movement' around a joint, and is vital for general mobility, including bending, lifting and reaching, and even walking and stair climbing. In the lower body, flexibility is particularly important around the hip joint and the hamstrings (the muscles at the back of the thighs). Well-stretched hamstrings can help avoid back pain and even how well we walk. In the upper body we need flexibility to comfortably comb our hair, fasten a back zip and for getting dressed. Even more importantly, poor upper body flexibility can result in a poor posture, leading to chronic neck and shoulder pain and balance problems, which in turn can lead to an increased risk of falling. And how do we become more flexible? By exercising and stretching after a workout – and at any time you feel like it.

Lower Body Flexibility Test

Equipment: a sturdy dining chair and a 12 inch ruler

- Sit on the edge of the chair with your preferred leg fully straightened out in line with the hip, with the heel on the floor
- The other leg is bent at 90 degrees with the foot flat on the floor.

273

- Overlap both hands with the middle fingers on top of each other and sit up before reaching as far as possible on the straight leg towards the toes.
- Practise twice first and then record the test. The aim is to reach as near to your toes as possible (or beyond), and then measure the distance between the tip of your fingers to the tip of your toes to the nearest half inch. It is a minus (−*inches*) score if your reach is *short* of the toes, and a plus (+*inches*) score if your reach goes *beyond* your toes.

Age Group	60+ F	M	70+ F	M	80+ F	M	90+ F	M
Excellent	+5	+3.5	+3.5	+2.5	+3.0	+1.5	+1.0	−0.5
Above Average	+3	+1.5	+2.5	+1	+1	−0.5	+0.5	−2.5
Average	+1.5	0.0	+1	−0.5	+0.5	−2.5	−2	−4
Below Average	0.0	−1.5	−0.5	−2.5	−1.5	−4.5	3.5	−5.5
Needs Practice	−2	−4.5	−1	−5	−3.5	−7	−6	−8

Upper Body Flexibility Test

Equipment: a 12 inch ruler

- Choose your most flexible side by putting one hand back over its same shoulder to see how far you can reach down (you can usually feel which side is more comfortable).
- With the hand over your shoulder and down your back, bend your other arm around and up your back, reaching toward the middle, toward the other hand, palms outward.

- Do 2 trial tests before measuring.
- Now measure the gap between the two middle fingers, or the length of the overlap.
- Record scores to the nearest half inch. *Minus* (–) scores represent the distance *short* of touching the middle fingers and *plus* (+) scores indicate the amount of *overlap* of the middle fingers.

Age Group	60+ F	M	70+ F	M	80+ F	M	90+ F	M
Excellent	+1.5	0	+1.0	–1	0	–2	–1	–4
Above Average	0	–2	–1	–3	–1.5	–4	–3	–6
Average	–1.5	–4	–2	–5	–3	6	–5	–8
Below Average	–2.5	–6	–3.5	–7	–4.5	–8.5	–7	–10
Needs Practice	–3	–8	–4	–10	–5	–11	–7.5	–12

Test 5

Balance Test

To move efficiently in everyday life, we need a good postural alignment and good balance. We can improve our balance significantly with regular practice in much the same way as doing exercises with weights improves our muscle strength. Poor balance greatly increases the risk of falling, which can have very serious consequences when we are older. Try this test and work towards improving your balance by practising 3–4 times per week.

Standing on One Leg (static)
Equipment: none

- In bare feet and on a hard floor, stand close to a wall or other surface so that you can hold on if necessary. Lift one foot off the floor and count the number of seconds you can balance, without holding on for support, before the foot has to be replaced.
- Do the same test with the other leg.

AGE-RELATED	TARGETS
UNDER 40	45 seconds
UNDER 60	40 seconds
AGED 60+	30 seconds
AGED 75+	20 seconds

Body Mass Index (BMI)

We have talked about our Body Mass Index (BMI) throughout this book. If we do need to lose weight, then knowing our BMI helps us to understand our level of overweight and its relevance and implications to our general health. It also helps us know where we need to be on the scales to be considered a 'healthy' weight.

BODY MASS INDEX – WHAT DOES IT MEAN?	
BMI LESS THAN 20	Underweight
BMI BETWEEN 20–24.9	Healthy Range
BMI BETWEEN 25–29.9	Overweight
BMI OVER 30	Obese
BMI OVER 40	Morbidly Obese

It is very easy to find out your BMI by going to the NHS website www.nhs.uk/bmicalculator and following the instructions. If you can, try to get an accurate confirmation of your current height because if you are in the older age group, there is a chance you are not as tall as you used to be.

11. Onwards and Upwards

I believe the coronavirus pandemic has given us all a very big wake-up call. The heartbreak has been unbearable, and the fear of contracting the virus has surely been felt by every single one of us. Across the whole world, lives will never be the same again.

Up to now many of us have taken our way of life for granted – travel and transportation, entertainment and employment, flying and dining, as well as holidays, hospitality and hospitals. Yes. Free healthcare to everyone in the UK since 1948. We had it all. And did we appreciate it? Absolutely not. Do we appreciate it now? You bet we do!

Our respect, appreciation, admiration, inspiration and total gratitude for our NHS is palpable. For everyone. The whole team – from cleaners to consultants, student nurses to surgeons, paramedics to care workers – we all take our hat off to them and say a massive THANK YOU!

I wonder whether we will ever be able to relax from the threat of COVID-19? It's probable we will only be able to do that when most people have been vaccinated and when testing is so sophisticated that we will know if we have come even close to someone who is affected. We are so grateful to all the scientists and technicians who are working so hard on our behalf. So many lessons are being learnt to enable us to be ready should another virus raise its ugly head in the future.

Time for action

So now it is over to us. It is time for us to take responsibility for our own health. If you are a smoker, now is the time to stop. If you drink too much alcohol, now is the time to cut back. If you are overweight, now is the time to make some serious changes to your eating habits and lose some weight. If you don't usually exercise, now is the time to get moving.

We have learnt the importance of social hygiene – keeping a social distance, washing hands thoroughly, using hand sanitisers, wearing a mask, and generally being much more cautious in our everyday lives. All of these actions can be life-saving and we should continue to use them until we are told we don't need to, but ensuring what we put inside our body is *healthy* rather than *harmful*, has to be our main priority. It just makes sense.

Hopefully, this Immunity Plan will have helped you to make some important lifestyle changes, which, if followed into the future, should significantly help you to survive if you do fall victim to this or any other virus, but perhaps just as importantly, by following the advice in this book, you will also have improved your general health and fitness, helping you to avoid heart disease, diabetes, some cancers and to live a significantly longer, fitter and happier life.

Enjoy the journey!

Sources

For further information, you may find the following academic papers helpful:

Schuch FB, Vancampfort D, Rosenbaum S, Richards J, Ward PB, Veronese N, Solmi M, Cadore EL, Stubbs B. **Exercise for Depression in Older Adults: a meta-analysis of randomized controlled trials adjusting for publication bias.** Braz J Psychiatry. 2016 Jul-Sep;38(3):247-54. doi: 10.1590/1516-4446-2016-1915. Epub 2016 Jul 18. PMID: 27611903; PMCID: PMC7194268.

Gschwind YJ, Kressig RW, Lacroix A, Muehlbauer T, Pfenninger B, Granacher U. **A Best Practice Fall Prevention Exercise Program to Improve Balance, Strength/Power, and Psychosocial Health in Older Adults: study protocol for a randomized controlled trial.** BMC Geriatr. 2013 Oct 9;13:105. doi: 10.1186/1471-2318-13-105. PMID: 24106864; PMCID: PMC3852637.

Belvederi Murri M, Amore M, Menchetti M, Toni G, Neviani F, Cerri M, Rocchi MB, Zocchi D, Bagnoli L, Tam E, Buffa A, Ferrara S, Neri M, Alexopoulos GS, Zanetidou S. **Safety and Efficacy of Exercise for Depression in Seniors (SEEDS) Study Group. Physical Exercise for Late-life Major Depression.** Br J Psychiatry. 2015 Sep;207(3):235-42. doi: 10.1192/bjp.bp.114.150516. Epub 2015 Jul 23. PMID: 26206864.

Aguiñaga S, Ehlers DK, Salerno EA, Fanning J, Motl RW, McAuley E. **Home-Based Physical Activity Program**

Improves Depression and Anxiety in Older Adults. J Phys Act Health. 2018 Sep 1;15(9):692-696. doi: 10.1123/jpah.2017-0390. Epub 2018 Apr 6. PMID: 29625012.

Breda J, Jewell J, Keller A. The Importance of the World Health Organization Sugar Guidelines for Dental Health and Obesity Prevention. Caries Res. 2019;53(2): 149-152. doi: 10.1159/000491556. Epub 2018 Aug 7. PMID: 30086553; PMCID: PMC6425811.

de Capo R, Mattson MP. Erratum for Effects of Intermittent Fasting on Health, Aging, and Disease. N Engl J Med. 2019 Dec 26;381(26):2541-2551. doi: 10.1056/NEJMra1905136. PMID: 31881139 Review. No abstract available.

1: Cueni LN, Detmar M. The Lymphatic System in Health and Disease. Lymphat Res Biol. 2008;6(3-4):109-22. doi: 10.1089/lrb.2008.1008. PMID: 19093783; PMCID: PMC3572233.

2: Liao S, von der Weid PY. Lymphatic System: An Active Pathway for Immune Protection. Semin Cell Dev Biol. 2015 Feb;38:83-9. doi: 10.1016/j.semcdb.2014.11.012. Epub 2014 Dec 19. PMID: 25534659; PMCID: PMC4397130.

3: Liao S, Padera TP. Lymphatic Function and Immune Regulation in Health and Disease. Lymphat Res Biol. 2013 Sep;11(3):136-43. doi: 10.1089/lrb.2013.0012. Epub 2013 Sep 11. PMID: 24024577; PMCID: PMC3780287.

Obrenovich ME, Li Y, Parvathaneni K, Yendluri BB, Palacios HH, Leszek J, Aliev G. Antioxidants in Health, Disease and Aging. CNS Neurol Disord Drug Targets. 2011 Mar;10(2): 192-207. doi: 10.2174/187152711794480375. PMID: 21226664.

Zolotukhin PV, Prazdnova EV, Chistyakov VA. Methods to Assess the Antioxidative Properties of Probiotics. Probiotics Antimicrob Proteins. 2018 Sep;10(3):589-599. doi: 10.1007/s12602-017-9375-6. PMID: 29249065.

Exercise training improves obesity-related lymphatic dysfunction.

Hespe GE, Kataru RP, Savetsky IL, García Nores GD, Torrisi JS, Nitti MD, Gardenier JC, Zhou J, Yu JZ, Jones LW, Mehrara BJ. J Physiol. 2016 Aug 1;594(15):4267-82. doi: 10.1113/JP271757. Epub 2016 Apr 9. PMID: 26931178. Free PMC article.

Items 1–3 of 3

1. The human gut microbiome as source of innovation for health: Which physiological and therapeutic outcomes could we expect?

Doré J, Multon MC, Béhier JM; participants of Giens XXXII, Round Table No. 2.
Therapie. 2017 Feb;72(1):21-38. doi: 10.1016/j.therap.2016.12.007. Epub 2017 Jan 3. PMID: 28131442

2. Gut-Joint Axis: The Role of Physical Exercise on Gut Microbiota Modulation in Older People with Osteoarthritis.

de Sire A, de Sire R, Petito V, Masi L, Cisari C, Gasbarrini A, Scaldaferri F, Invernizzi M.
Nutrients. 2020 Feb 22;12(2):574. doi: 10.3390/nu12020574. PMID: 32098380. Free PMC article. Review.

3. Prospective study of probiotic supplementation results in immune stimulation and improvement of upper respiratory infection rate.

Zhang H, Yeh C, Jin Z, Ding L, Liu BY, Zhang L, Dannelly HK. Synth Syst Biotechnol. 2018 Mar 12;3(2):113-120. doi: 10.1016/j. synbio.2018.03.001. eCollection 2018 Jun. PMID: 29900424. Free PMC article.

Acknowledgements

When we were celebrating the arrival of a new decade with a glass of bubbly, who would have believed what 2020 would throw at us? It was unimaginable that a virulent virus would make such a dramatic impact – not just on *our* lives, but across the whole world!

Toward the end of March my doctor called me. I have long-standing chest problems, so I was being advised to self-isolate for at least three months, possibly six. I knew that it was critical to my survival that I stayed safe, so there was no argument in my mind. As I prepared myself mentally, I decided to write a book to help the older generation to stay fit and healthy as I was now in that category.

I called my literary agent, Luigi Bonomi, and put the idea to him, but Luigi explained that publishers were looking for a small book that could be turned around fast and published as an eBook, based on becoming healthier during the pandemic. I immediately set to work. I also called my friend and colleague of 25 years, Mary Morris, to ask if she would like to be involved and ideally create a progressive workout for the older generation or for those who are not very fit. Thankfully, Mary was up for the challenge too.

Writing this book has been rewarding for both of us on so many levels. We have enjoyed learning about how we can help our immune system be the most effective it can be. We have also been happy to do something constructive and positive during our many lockdown months, and to produce something that hopefully will help others transform their lives and live longer.

So, as you can see, from the very start this has been a wonderful team effort. I am very grateful to Luigi for securing our wonderful publisher, Penguin. Once I was introduced to my Commissioning Editor, Ione Walder, and my Book Editor, Beatrix McIntyre, I knew this was going to be fun. Thank you all so much for your positivity and encouragement.

A very important part of the creation of this book is down to our wonderful trialists, who put the Plan to the test and produced the most amazing results and feedback that went way beyond what we expected. A heartfelt 'Thank You' to you all from Mary and from me for your efforts, diligence and remarkably positive results!

Thanks must also go to Penguin's Press Officer, Sriya Varadharajan, who secured some great interviews and press coverage for me. The radio chats were such fun and certainly boosted the sales of the original eBook, the direct result of which led to the publication of this extended version in paperback.

I must thank my PA, Peter Legg, for his help in so many ways, and to my husband, Mike, for his help and support throughout the writing of this book and in promoting it on social media on my behalf.

Most of all a massive thank you to Mary for her amazing contribution, hard work and constant enthusiasm and encouragement in making this book the best it could be. Her workouts and the Fitness Test have added something really special, which will make it so effective for everyone who follows it. And, of course, a huge thank you to Penguin for publishing this book for us.

Progress Charts

Weight and Inch Loss Record Chart

DATE	CURRENT WEIGHT	WEIGHT LOSS THIS WEEK	WEIGHT LOSS TO DATE	WAIST INCHES/CM	INCHES/CM LOSS TO DATE	NOTES

Fitness Test Progress Chart

DATE **BMI**											
SIT TO STAND (No. of Reps)											
ARM CURLS (No. of Reps)											
2-MINUTE STEP **TEST** (No. of Steps)											
SEATED REACH (+/− Inches/cm)											
BACK HAND **REACH** (+/− Inches/cm)											
BALANCE (No. of Seconds)	L	R	L	R	L	R	L	R	L	R	L	R

Favourite Recipes

NAME OF RECIPE	PAGE NO.

Rosemary's Participants After Completing The 28-Day Plan

Lesley

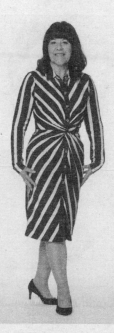

'I realise that as a society we are going through a terrible time, I used this time to do something positive to improve *my* life as I approach my 60s, and with the sacrifices we are all making to keep each other safe, I feel this has been so worth it. People often lose weight when they have a medical scare, but COVID-19 has presented us with the best "medical motivation" we could have. Let's not waste it.' *(Lesley lost 1 stone 7lbs over-all and now has a healthy BMI of 23.1)*

Brigitte

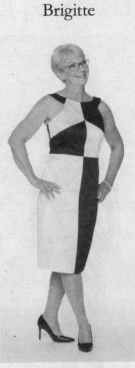

'I will recommend this Plan to anyone to make them feel good about themselves again. The biggest thing personally is that I never came across any negatives. The whole experience has given me a real boost and a wake-up call! Thank you for getting me back into a really healthy lifestyle!' *(Brigitte now has a healthy BMI of 22.3)*

Helen

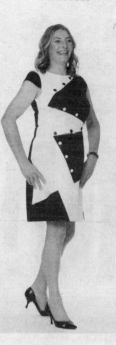

'Mentally I feel so much healthier, I am happier in myself and I know my confidence has increased. I now walk tall and stride out, with my head held high. I feel like a new me and I'm very proud of myself!'
(Helen lost a stone overall and now has a healthy BMI of 23)

Jennie and Kevin

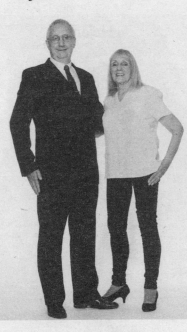

'Because of some stressful situations that I have had to deal with during lockdown, I feel that the fact that we have eaten healthily, and that I am so much fitter with more stamina, I have coped much better with stress during the difficult days.' *(Kevin lost 1 stone 4lbs and only needs to lose a little more to be able to fall into the 'healthy' BMI range)*

'I've enjoyed my daily walks with my son Kevin, and we have enjoyed cooking the different recipes from the Plan together. It has been helpful doing the Trial together and we are really pleased with how we have each lost over a stone. I have much more energy and confidence, which is a real bonus. I'm sleeping better too.' *(Jennie lost 1 stone 4lbs on the Plan and now has a healthy BMI of 22.1)*

Mike

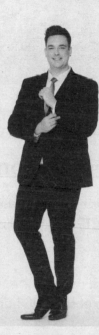

'I'm really happy that I have lost even more weight than I lost during the 28-day Trial. I have now joined a gym for the first time in a few years, which I feel is a really positive result emerging from doing the Trial. I realise I need to push myself a bit further and pick up the slack, so joining the gym is a really important step for me and now I have the confidence to do it.' *(Mike Coughlan lost 10lbs during the Trial)*

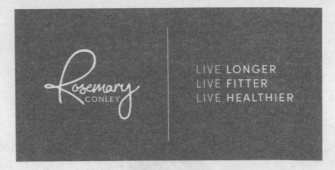

Coming soon in early 2021 the all new

www.rosemaryconley.com

This brand new website from Rosemary Conley CBE
gives FREE advice to help you:

- Boost your immune system
- Stay fitter into older age
- Learn from the experts including physiotherapists
  and specialists
- Cope with arthritis
- Stay young as you get older
- Get fit for an operation and speed up your
  recovery
- Cook delicious healthy food
- Find exercises you can do

www.rosemaryconley.com ~

HELPING YOU TO LIVE LONGER, FITTER AND HEALTHIER!